QBASE SURGERY: 1

MCQs FOR THE MRCS

QBASE SURGERY: 1

MCQs FOR THE MRCS

JSA Green LLM FRCS
Specialist Registrar in Urology
North Thames Deanery
London, UK

SA Wajed MA FRCS
Research Fellow, Department of Surgery
University of Southern California
Los Angeles, USA

QBase series developed and edited by

Edward J. Hammond MA BM BCh MRCP FRCA
Shackleton Department of Anaesthetics
Southampton University Hospital NHS Trust

Andrew K. McIndoe MC ChB FRCA
Sir Humphry Davy Department of Anaesthesia
Bristol Royal Infirmary

GMM

© 2001
Greenwich Medical Media Ltd.
137 Euston Road
London
NW1 2AA

ISBN 1 900151 37 5

First Published 2001

A catalogue record for this book is available from the British Library

Produced and Designed by
Saxon Graphics Limited, Derby

Printed in Great Britain

CONTENTS

Preface

Surgical training in the United Kingdom has undergone major structural changes in the last few years and is still continuing to evolve. This has been reflected in the transformation of the old fellowship examinations to the new MRCS syllabus. There has been a shift of emphasis from the traditional tests of surgical knowledge and operative skill to an understanding of the principles and systems of surgery. This is outlined for example in the new MRCS syllabus for the Royal College of Surgeons of England. This is split into a total of ten modules, five of which relate to the principles of surgery, and five which relate to the systems of surgery.

The method of examination, which formally included essays and short answers has been simplified to multiple choice questions of which again there are two papers testing principles and systems respectively. In addition, a further change has abolished the use of the negative marking system for incorrect responses.

MCQ's are designed to test a greater breadth of knowledge over an examination, and the depth of the understanding of an area can also be similarly adjusted. However, it takes away the means of expression, and the ability to justify an understanding of a topic which is more than merely factual. The loss of negative marking, which previously acted as a severe deterrent to guessing, now possibly encourages this strategy. The result is likely to mean a more narrow spread of results following the examination, and therefore a higher threshold of pass if standards are to be maintained.

This book and its free CD-ROM attempts to cover both the principles and systems of surgery with regard to the syllabuses of the four colleges of surgeons in the United Kingdom. The exams in all of these colleges are still undergoing adaptation and both the subject material and the breadth and depth of questioning is likely to continue to change over the next few years. It is hoped that the questions in this book and CD-ROM will provide an accurate representation of the MCQ exams and reflect the success a candidate is likely to be able to achieve. We intend to adapt this in the future to parallel the exams as closely as possible.

The key to success in answering MCQ's correctly is firstly to read and understand the meaning and phraseology of the question stem. This should then be repeated for each response to confirm that the statement makes sense. This will reduce the chance of an incorrect response due to ambiguity in the structure of the question. There are a number of terms which are commonly used in MCQ's, a summary of which is provided below. Finally, remember that there is also a time limit on the exam, and try not to spend more than the allocated time on each question as this will compromise your ability to understand clearly the later questions.

Wishing you the best of luck.

James Green
Saj Wajed
London and Los Angeles
July 2000

COMMON MCQ TERMINOLOGY

Characteristic, classical, predominantly, reliably	At least 90% of cases
Typically, frequently, commonly, usually	At least 60% of cases
Often, tends to	At least 30% of cases
Has been shown, associated, recognised	Evidence in recognised publication
Immediate	Within 3 hours
Urgent	Within 24 hours

RUNNING THE QBASE
PROGRAM ON CD-ROM

SYSTEM REQUIREMENTS

An IBM compatible PC with a minimum 80386 processor and 4MB of RAM VGA Monitor set up to display at least 256 colours.

CD-ROM drive

Windows 3.1 or higher with Microsoft compatible mouse

The display setting of your computer must be set to display "SMALL FONTS".

See Windows manuals for further instructions on how to do this.

INSTALLATION INSTRUCTIONS

The program will install the appropriate files onto you hard drive. It requires the QBase CD-ROM to be installed in the D:\drive.

In order to run QBase the CD-ROM must be in the drive.

Print Readme.txt and Helpfile.txt on the CD-ROM for fuller instructions and user manual

Windows 95/98

1. Insert the QBase CD-ROM into drive D:

2. From the **Start Menu**, select the RUN **option**

3. Type **D:\setup.exe and press enter or return**

4. **Follow the Full Installation** option and accept the default directory for installation of QBase.

   The installation program creates a folder called **QBase** containing the program icon and another called **Exams** into which you can save previous exam attempts.

5. To run QBase double click the **QBase** icon in the QBase folder. From windows Explorer double click the **QBase.exe** file in the QBase folder.

Windows 3.1/Windows for Workgroups 3.11

1. Insert the QBase CD-ROM into the drive D:

2. From the **File Menu**, select the **RUN option**

3. Type **D:\setup.exe and press enter or return**

4. Follow the instruction given by the installation program. Select the **Full Installation** option and accept the default directory for installation of QBase

   The Installation program creates a program window and directory called **QBase** containing the program icon. It also creates a directory called **Exams** into which you can save previous attempts.

5. To run QBase double click on the **QBase** icon in the QBase program. From File Manager double click the **QBase.exe** file in the QBase directory.

Exam 1

QUESTION 1

Patients with very high alcohol intake undergoing surgery

- **A.** Require smaller doses of sedation and anaesthesia
- **B.** Have an increased incidence of deep vein thrombosis
- **C.** Have an increased risk of wound infection
- **D.** Have an increased risk of post-operative confusion
- **E.** Have increased risk of cardiac complications

QUESTION 2

A chest radiograph

- **A.** Should be taken PA (posterior-anterior) if possible
- **B.** Is often normal in pulmonary embolism
- **C.** Shows left sided mediastinal shift in aortic dissection
- **D.** Shows Kerley B lines in association with a tension pneumothorax
- **E.** Show plethoric lung fields in the presence of a left to right shunt

QUESTION 3

Children under five years old undergoing minor surgery with a general anaesthetic

- **A.** Can be fed an hour before surgery
- **B.** Normally do not require blood tests if previously fit and well
- **C.** Can be suitable for day surgery
- **D.** Should be given pre-operative heparin
- **E.** Do require a routine chest X-ray

QUESTION 4

Drugs used in pre-medication for anaesthesia prior to surgery

- **A.** Metoclopromide reduces risk of reflux
- **B.** Benzodiazepines reduce salivary secretions
- **C.** Phenothiazines act against GABA receptors
- **D.** Promethiazine can act as a bronchodilator
- **E.** Opiods can cause bronchoconstriction

QUESTION 5

Hypoxaemia

A. Occurs when the PaO_2 is less than 9 kPa
B. Is always associated with a rise in $PaCO_2$
C. May occur in Adult Respiratory Distress Syndrome (ARDS)
D. May occur in acute pulmonary embolism
E. Is associated with acidosis

QUESTION 6

Tourniquets for isolated limb surgery

A. Should only be used in conjunction with a general anaesthetic
B. The cuff is normally inflated to 70-100 mmHg in the lower limb
C. Are contraindicated in sickle cell disease
D. Are contraindicated in peripheral vascular disease
E. There may be a rise in serum potassium after deflation

QUESTION 7

Massive blood transfusions are associated with

A. Hyperkalaemia
B. Hypercalcaemia
C. Hypothermia
D. Hypercoagulabity
E. Haemolytic jaundice

QUESTION 8

Causes of a decreased urine output in a gastrectomy patient six hours post operatively include

A. Blocked catheter
B. Third space sequestration
C. Pulmonary oedema
D. Inadequate fluid replacement
E. Glomerulonephritis

QUESTION 9

Regarding cardiac arrhythmia

A. Ventricular ectopics at a rate of less than 8/min are not regarded as significant
B. Sinus bradycardia may be precipitated by pharyngeal suction
C. Sinus tachycardia results in decreased coronary artery perfusion
D. Atrial fibrillation may be treated with adenosine infusions
E. Are sensitive to serum potassium

QUESTION 10

Surgical instruments may be sterilised by

A. Gamma irradiation
B. Glutaraldehyde
C. Ethylene oxide
D. Boiling water
E. Hot air

QUESTION 11

Risk of post operative wound infection is increased by

A. Local ischaemia
B. Post-operative haematoma
C. Jaundice
D. Malnutrition
E. Uraemia

QUESTION 12

Monopolar diathermy

A. Uses alternating current at 50 Hz
B. Requires the use of an earthing plate
C. Can be used for cutting if the output is pulsed
D. Can be safely used on extremities
E. Can transmit current along any metal instrument

QUESTION 13

Factors associated with poor wound healing include

A. Vitamin A deficiency
B. Vitamin B1 deficiency
C. Vitamin C deficiency
D. Folate deficiency
E. Zinc deficiency

QUESTION 14

Damage to the following nerves is a recognised complication during these procedures

A. Ilioinguinal nerve and inguinal hernia mesh repair
B. Axillary nerve and axillary clearance
C. Sciatic nerve and posterior approach total hip replacement
D. Facial nerve and parotidectomey
E. Lateral popliteal nerve and short saphenous vein ligation

QUESTION 15

Diagnostic peritoneal lavage (DPL)

A. Involves the installation of warm saline into the peritoneal cavity
B. Should be done under general anaesthetic
C. Is "positive" if bowel contents are found in the aspirate
D. Should not be performed in unstable patients or those with multiple injuries
E. Is contraindicated in pregnancy

QUESTION 16

During the "acute" or "ebb" phase in the physiological response to injury

A. Anti-Diuretic Hormone is secreted from the hypothalamus into circulation which increases retention of water
B. There is a rise in the level of circulating fatty acids due to increased mobilisation and reduced uptake by tissues
C. Insulin levels rise in response to adrenergic activity on the pancreas
D. Plasma proteins including CRP and fibrinogen are raised
E. ACTH is secreted in large amounts from the adrenal glands

QUESTION 17

The following viruses have been associated with malignancies below

A. Hepatitis C virus and hepatocellular carcinoma of the liver
B. Epstein–Barr virus and nasopharyngeal cancer
C. Human T-cell leukaemia virus type I (HTLV-1) and Burkitt's lymphoma
D. Human papilloma virus (HPV) and endometrial carcinoma
E. Human Immunodeficiency virus (HIV) and adenocarcinoma of the rectum

QUESTION 18

The following cytoplasmic oncogenes have been linked with the malignancies below

A. erb-B2 and prostate cancer
B. ras and malignant melanoma
C. int-2 and pancreatic carcinoma
D. abl and ovarian cancer
E. sis and colorectal cancer

QUESTION 19

Malignant melanoma

A. Is the most common skin cancer in the UK
B. The Lentigo maligna type has a poor prognosis
C. A lesion between 0.76 - 1.5 mm thick indicates a 50% chance of lymph node involvement
D. A lesion greater than 3.0 mm deep will require an excision margin of at least 50mm
E. Extension into the subcutaneous fat (Clark's level V) give a five year survival rate of 15-30%

QUESTION 20

Hypersplenism can occur in

A. Malaria
B. Gaucher's disease
C. Chronic Lymphoid leukaemia
D. Cystic Fibrosis
E. Rheumatoid arthritis

QUESTION 21

The major histocompatibilty complex antigens (MHC antigens)

A. Are all located on chromosome 6
B. Type I antigens are present on all cells
C. Type I are coded for on three loci A, B and C
D. Type II are coded on three loci DR, DQ and DP
E. Matching HLA genes is essential for graft survival in liver transplantation

QUESTION 22

The following drugs may exacerbate a bleeding tendency

A. Cimetidine
B. Voltarol
C. Metronidazole
D. Oral contraceptive pill
E. Gentamicin

QUESTION 23

Complications of introducing a Swann–Ganz catheter include

A. Dysrhythmia during insertion
B. Pulmonary infarction
C. Atelectasis
D. Bacterial endocarditis
E. Pneumonia

QUESTION 24

The coroner is normally informed in the following situations

A. Death in a HIV positive patient
B. Death within 24 hours of admission to hospital
C. Death on the operating table
D. Death following an alleged violent incident
E. Death following attempted suicide

QUESTION   25

The third cranial nerve (oculomotor nerve)

A. Arises from the pons
B. Runs between the superior cerebellar and posterior cerebral arteries
C. Enters the orbit via the superior orbital fissure
D. Supplies all the orbital muscles with the exception of the lateral rectus
E. Paralysis results in loss of accommodation and reaction to light

QUESTION   26

Tumours of the anterior pituitary gland

A. Are very rarely malignant
B. Can cause a bi-temporal hemianopia
C. Can secrete cortisol causing Cushing's disease
D. Can secrete ADH causing water retention
E. Can secrete prolactin causing amenorrhoea in women

QUESTION   27

Nasopharyngeal cancer

A. May present with major epistaxis
B. Is associated with the Epstein-Barr virus
C. Radiotherapy is the first line treatment
D. Lymph node spread ocurs firs to the anterior triange
E. Is an adenocarcinoma

QUESTION   28

Symptoms of a primary lung cancer can include

A. Hoarse voice
B. Haemoptysis
C. Leuconychia
D. Finger clubbing
E. Dysphagia

QUESTION   29

Coarctation of the aorta

A. The commonest site for stenosis is just distal to the origin of the left subclavian artery
B. In the adult is associated with a patent ductus arteriosus in the majority of cases
C. In the infant, is associated with cyanosis of the lower limbs
D. May present with intermittent claudication
E. Rib notching is commonly seen in the chest x-rays in young children

QUESTION 30

Atheromatous disease in the aorto–iliac region

A. Is not usually amenable to successful angioplasty
B. Claudication pain can be felt in the buttocks
C. May present as impotence
D. Femoral pulses are usually normal
E. Collateral vessels rarely develop

QUESTION 31

Abdominal aortic aneurysms

A. Have an operative mortality of over 50% following acute rupture
B. Have a operative mortality of over 10% if operated electively
C. Can present with symptoms of sciatica alone
D. Surgery should be considered for aneurysm of 5.5cm or greater maximal diameter on ultrasound
E. Extend above the renal vessels in 5% of cases

QUESTION 32

Causes of chronic lower limb ulcers include

A. Rheumatoid arthritis
B. Diabetes mellitus
C. Lymhoedema
D. Melanoma
E. Osteomylitis

QUESTION 33

Plain X-ray features of osteoarthritis include

A. Narrowing of the joint space
B. Subarticular sclerosis
C. Decreased trabecular pattern
D. Subchondral bone cyst formation
E. Osteophyte formation

QUESTION 34

Causes of osteoporosis include

A. Hyperparathyroidism
B. High alcohol intake
C. Cushing's disease
D. Hypothyroidism
E. Scurvy

QUESTION   35

Avascular necrosis is a recognised complication of the following fractures

A. Mid-shaft femoral
B. Distal radial
C. Tri-malleolar
D. Scaphoid
E. Femoral neck

QUESTION   36

Ranson criteria for severe pancreatitis include

A. Age over 65 years
B. WBC greater than16 000 mm^3 on admission
C. Serum AST (aspartate transaminase) over 250 IU/l on admission
D. Rise in haematocrit of above 10 during the initial 48 hours
E. PaCO$_2$ greater than 5 kPa after 48 hours

QUESTION   37

Factors which may cause acute pancreatitis include

A. Endoscopic retrograde cholangio-pancreatography (ERCP)
B. Mesenteric ischaemia
C. Gallstones
D. Peptic Ulcer disease
E. Trauma

QUESTION   38

Gallstones

A. Are more common in women
B. Are commonly radiologically lucent
C. Large solitary stones are composed of calcium bilirubinate
D. Impacted in the cystic duct can cause obstructive jaundice
E. In the presence of colonic diverticular disease an peptic ulcer disease is known as Saint's triad

QUESTION   39

Stilboestrol (phosphorylated diethlstilboestrol)

A. May cause gynaecomastia
B. Is a luteinising hormone releasing hormone analogue
C. Is given by a monthly depot
D. Is used in the treatement of benign prostatic hypertrophy
E. Can cause thromboembolic problems

QUESTION 40

Carcinoma of the bladder

A. Is most commonly an adenocarcinoma
B. The most common site of occurrence is in the bladder neck
C. The most common presentation is retention of urine
D. In the TNM staging, T3 indicates involvement of the full thickness of the muscle wall
E. Intravesical chemotherapy using BCG is effective in reducing the recurrence rate

QUESTION 41

Testicular tumours

A. Are a feature of older men
B. The tumor marker alpha-feto-protein (AFP) is often raised
C. Spread usually occurs to inguinal nodes
D. Do not respond to radiotherapy
E. Metastatic disease is treated with palladium based chemotherapy

QUESTION 42

Hypercalcaemia can occur in

A. Chronic renal failure
B. Breast cancer
C. Myelofibrosis
D. Follicular carcinoma of the thyroid
E. Sarcoidosis

QUESTION 43

The following are clinical features of thyrotoxicosis

A. Cardiac arrythmias
B. Irritability
C. Amenorrhoea
D. Alopecia
E. Vitiligo

QUESTION 44

Zollinger-Ellison syndrome

A. Is usually due to a tumour of the G cells within the pancreas
B. Presents with widespread peptic ulceration
C. Can be associated with raised levels of parathormone (PTH)
D. Raised serum secretin levels are diagnostic
E. Is treated with primary systemic chemotherapy

QUESTION 45

The female breast

A. Is an ectodermal in embryological origin
B. Can arise anywhere along the "milk line" from the axillae to the umbilicus resulting in accessory breasts
C. Receives blood supply from perforating branches of the internal thoracic artery
D. Overlies the pectoralis major, serratus anterior and rectus sheath
E. Over 90% of the lymphatic drainage occurs through the ipsilateral axilla

QUESTION 46

In the TNM staging of breast cancer

A. T2 indicates the primary tumour is less than 2 cm greatest diameter
B. Peau d'orange qualifies for T4 classification
C. N2 indicates involvement of ipsilateral internal mammary nodes
D. Pagets disease equates to a T1 lesion
E. Supraclavicular node involvement is regarded as M1

QUESTION 47

Male breast cancer

A. The lobular variety is most common
B. Occurs more commonly in younger men
C. Risk may be increased in Turner's syndrome
D. Radical radiotherapy is the treatment of choice
E. Tumours do not normally respond to tamoxifen

QUESTION 48

Persistant, conjugated hyperbilirubinaemia may be caused by

A. Alpha-1-antitrypsin deficiency
B. Hypothyroidism
C. Haemolytic disease
D. Cytomegalovirus infection
E. Cystic fibrosis

QUESTION 49

Medical conditions that can mimic an acute surgical abdomen include

A. Pneumonia
B. Diabetes insipidus
C. Sickle cell disease
D. Haemolytic uraemic syndrome
E. Dandy–Walker syndrome

QUESTION   50

Circumcision of the male penis is indicated in the following clinical situations

A. Hypospadias
B. Balanitis xerotica obliterans
C. Non-retractile foreskin in neonates
D. Recurrent paraphimosis
E. Posterior urethral valve

Exam 1: Answers

QUESTION 1

A. FALSE B. FALSE C. TRUE D. TRUE E. TRUE

Alcohol dependant patients have high tolerance to anaesthetic agents. There may be associated hepatic, cardiac and cerebral damage.

QUESTION 2

A. TRUE B. TRUE C. FALSE D. FALSE E. TRUE

AP Chest X-rays are only taken if the patient is unable to stand up. The definition of the cardiac border is not as clear as in a PA view. Pulmonary embolism only rarely shows abnormalities on a chest X-ray. Widening of the mediastinum is seen in aortic dissection, and Kerley B lines are associated with pulmonary oedema.

QUESTION 3

A. FALSE B. TRUE C. TRUE D. FALSE E. FALSE

Day surgery is suitable for children whose parents or guardians are able to take responsibility for care. For minor surgery no routine investigations are warranted. Feeding is normally suspended at least four hours pre-operatively, though practice may vary.

QUESTION 4

A. TRUE B. FALSE C. FALSE D. TRUE E. TRUE

Benzodiazepines (e.g. temazepam) are anxiolytics and sedatives which act on GABA receptors. They have no effect on secretions. Phenothiazines act against DOPA, cholinergic and histamine receptors, resulting in axiolysis, sedation, and antiemesis as well as bronchodilation. Metoclopromide increases gastric motility and oesophageal sphincter pressure, reducing reflux as well as being an anti-emetic. Opioids are good analgesics but side effects include nausea, vomiting and bronchospasm.

QUESTION 5

A. TRUE B. FALSE C. TRUE D. TRUE E. FALSE

Hypoxaemia is a low oxygenation of arterial blood, and is due to inadaquate oxygenation, hypoventilation or ventilation perfusion mismatch. Providing CO_2 is not retained (ventilatory failure), hypercapnia and respiratory acidosis will not occur.

QUESTION 6

A. FALSE   B. FALSE   C. TRUE   D. TRUE   E. TRUE

Padded tourniquets can be used for applying a local block or "blood-free" surgery. In the upper limb, it is inflated to 30-50 mmHg above systolic pressure, and 70-100 mmHg above systolic pressure in the lower limb. Post deflation, there is a release of anaerobic metabolites and reactive hyperaemia.

QUESTION 7

A. TRUE   B. FALSE   C. TRUE   D. FALSE   E. TRUE

Blood is stored at 4°C in the form of packed cells, and with added citrate. This chelates calcium and depletes clotting factors. Lysis of cells releases potassium.

QUESTION 8

A. TRUE   B. FALSE   C. FALSE   D. TRUE   E. FALSE

Urine output falls following trauma or surgery as part of a stress reaction. Inadequate fluid maintenance is the most common cause of persistently low urine output.

QUESTION 9

A. FALSE   B. TRUE   C. TRUE   D. FALSE   E. TRUE

Ventricular ectopics over 6/min are regarded as significant. Pharyngeal stimulation during suction may result in vagal activity. Increased rate reduces diastolic time and hence coronary artery perfusion. Correction of electrolytes, fluid balance and oxygenation reduce the chance of arrhythmia developing.

QUESTION 10

A. TRUE   B. TRUE   C. TRUE   D. FALSE   E. TRUE

Heat sterilisation uses pressured steam or hot air to achieve temperatures over 120°C.

QUESTION 11

A. TRUE   B. TRUE   C. TRUE   D. TRUE   E. TRUE

Local and systemic factors apply to the healing of tissues.

QUESTION 12

A. FALSE   B. TRUE   C. FALSE   D. FALSE   E. TRUE

Diathermy uses alternating current at frequencies over 50 000 Hz (50 kHz). Monopolar diathermy transmits current through the patient via a plate, the area of highest current concentration being diathermied.

QUESTION 13

A. TRUE   B. FALSE   C. TRUE   D. FALSE   E. TRUE

QUESTION   14

A. TRUE   B. FALSE   C. TRUE   D. TRUE   E. TRUE

The thoracodorsal and long thoracic nerves are at risk in an axillary clearance

QUESTION   15

A. TRUE   B. FALSE   C. TRUE   D. FALSE   E. TRUE

DPL is a crude but quick way to assess the possibility of an intra-abdominal bleed in cases where the patient is to unwell to have a CT scan or it is not available. A positive test indicates need for urgent laparotomy, which in up to 30% of cases has proven to be unnecessary.

QUESTION   16

A. FALSE   B. TRUE   C. FALSE   D. TRUE   E. FALSE

ACTH (anterior pituitary) and ADH (posterior pituitary) are released along with catecholamines as part of the hormonal response to injury. Plasma, glucose, fatty acids and proteins are all raised , and insulin secretion is suppressed.

QUESTION   17

A. FALSE   B. TRUE   C. FALSE   D. FALSE   E. FALSE

Hepatitis B virus is associated with carcinoma of the liver. EBV is associated with both nasopharyngeal carcinoma and Burkitt's lymphoma. HPV and HIV have both been linked to cervical cancer.

QUESTION   18

A. FALSE   B. FALSE   C. FALSE   D. FALSE   E. FALSE

Weak association between ras, erb-B2 , abl and carcinoma of the colon, breast and leukaemia have been reported.

QUESTION   19

A. FALSE   B. FALSE   C. FALSE   D. TRUE   E. TRUE

Malignant melanoma is the least common skin cancer but has a high malignant potential and spreads via lymph nodes and blood. The disease is classified using the Breslow (thickness of lesion) or Clark's level of invasion methods which give an indication of lymph node involvement and prognosis.

QUESTION   20

A. TRUE   B. TRUE   C. TRUE   D. FALSE   E. TRUE

Hypersplenism is splenomegaly associated with reduced numbers of circulating blood cells of at least one type.

QUESTION 21

A. TRUE   B. TRUE   C. TRUE   D. TRUE   E. FALSE

Good HLA matching is important in renal transplantation, giving a one year survival rate of over 90%. In liver transplantation, ABO match is normally sufficient.

QUESTION 22

A. TRUE   B. TRUE   C. TRUE   D. FALSE   E. FALSE

The oral contraceptive pill predisposes to thrombosis. The other drugs can potentiate the effect of warfarin.

QUESTION 23

A. TRUE   B. FALSE   C. FALSE   D. TRUE   E. FALSE

A Swann-Ganz catheter is a balloon tipped catheter which is wedged within a small branch of the pulmonary artery and gives a good guide to the left atrial pressure. This is called the pulmonary capillary wedge pressure (PCWP).

QUESTION 24

A. FALSE   B. TRUE   C. TRUE   D. FALSE   E. TRUE

Any death which occurs in strange or unexpected circumstances must be reported to the coroner who then decides whether a post-mortem and or inquest is to be made.

QUESTION 25

A. FALSE   B. TRUE   C. TRUE   D. FALSE   E. TRUE

The third nerve arises from the midbrain, the nucleus lying in the floor of the aqueduct of Sylvius. It supplies the ciliary ganglion with parasympathetic fibres necessary for pupillary constriction, and all the external ocular muscles except superior oblique and lateral rectus.

QUESTION 26

A. TRUE   B. TRUE   C. FALSE   D. FALSE   E. TRUE

Pituitary tumours are usually adenomas, and can arise from any of the six hormone secreting cells. The hormones produced are TSH, GH. Prolactin, ACTH, and the gonadotrophins LH and FSH. Pressure on the optic nerve interferes with the decussating fibres at the optic chiasm first. ADH is a posterior pituitary hormone.

QUESTION 27

A. FALSE   B. TRUE   C. TRUE   D. FALSE   E. FALSE

Nasopharyngeal carcinoma is common in oriental countries. It presents with serous nasal discharge or obstruction, serous aural discharge or hearing problems or diplopia due to abducens nerve involvement. Most tumours are radiosensitive. Lymph nodes palpable in the posterior triangle may be the first presentation. The lesion is squamous cell.

QUESTION   28

A. TRUE   B. TRUE   C. FALSE   D. TRUE   E. TRUE

Local invasion of structures, including the recurrent Laryngeal nerve, and oesophagus can give rise to voice changes and dysphagia respectively. Clubbing is associated with pulmonary osteoarthropathy.

QUESTION   29

A. TRUE   B. FALSE   C. TRUE   D. TRUE   E. FALSE

In coarctation of the aorta the stenosis is most common just beyond the origin of the left subclavian artery. In adults there is a patent ductus arteriosus in a minority of cases, but in the infant this can cause a differential cyanosis of the lower limbs. Reduced perfusion of the lower limbs can give rise to intermittent claudication. Rib notching is a common feature in adult chest X-rays.

QUESTION   30

A. FALSE   B. TRUE   C. TRUE   D. FALSE   E. FALSE

Leriche's syndrome is the combination of male impotence with occlusive disease in the region of the aortic bifurcation. Femoral pulses are weak or absent, but there can be good collateral development.

QUESTION   31

A. TRUE   B. FALSE   C. TRUE   D. TRUE   E. TRUE

Acute rupture is associated with a high mortality. This can be lowered to less than 5% if managed electively. A maximal diameter of greater than 5.5 cm exponentially increases the risks of rupture.

QUESTION   32

A. TRUE   B. TRUE   C. TRUE   D. TRUE   E. TRUE

The most common cause of chronic lower limb ulcers is venous insufficiency, followed by arterial disease.

QUESTION   33

A. FALSE   B. TRUE   C. FALSE   D. TRUE   E. TRUE

Osteopenia may also result due to decreased use.

QUESTION   34

A. TRUE   B. TRUE   C. TRUE   D. FALSE   E. TRUE

Osteoporosis is reduced bone per unit volume, but is qualitatively normal. It can also occur in thyrotoxicosis.

QUESTION   35

A. FALSE   B. FALSE   C. FALSE   D. TRUE   E. TRUE

Avascular necrosis is a possibility if the blood supply to a region is compromised following fracture.

QUESTION   36

A. FALSE   B. TRUE   C. TRUE   D. TRUE   E. FALSE

Age over 55 is a severe prognostic factor. $PaCO_2$ is not used in severity scores.

QUESTION   37

A. TRUE   B. TRUE   C. TRUE   D. FALSE   E. TRUE

The most common causes of pancreatitis are alcohol and gallstones. Peptic Ulcer disease and mesenteic ischaemia can cause hyperamylasemia.

QUESTION   38

A. TRUE   B. TRUE   C. FALSE   D. TRUE   E. FALSE

Gallstones have a higher incidence in women. The majority are mixed, but 95% contain cholesterol. Pure cholesterol stones can form large solitary lesions. Pigment stones are small and faceted, and are composed of calcium bilrubinate. Only 10% are seen on plain X-rays. In Mirrizzi syndrome, a stone in the cystic duct can cause localised pressure on the common bile duct causing jaundice. Saint's triad consists of gallstones, diverticular disease and hiatus hernia.

QUESTION   39

A. TRUE   B. FALSE   C. FALSE   D. FALSE   E. TRUE

Stilboestrol is used in the hormonal treatment of prostatic cancer. Side effects include loss of libido, gynaecomastia, heart failure, and cerebrovascular accidents. It is a testosterone inhibiting drug and is normally taken orally.

QUESTION   40

A. FALSE   B. FALSE   C. FALSE   D. TRUE   E. TRUE

Transitional cell carcinoma is the most common form in England. In areas where Schistosomiasis is present, squamous cell carcinoma is common. Most lesions occur in the trigone and lateral walls. Painless haematuria is the typical presentation.

QUESTION   41

A. FALSE   B. TRUE   C. FALSE   D. FALSE   E. FALSE

Testicular tumours occur in young men, with teratomas occurring in the late teens, and seminomas in the early 30's. Tumour markers AFP and β-HCG are raised and are later used to monitor the disease. Spread occurs to the para-aortic lymph nodes. Seminoma are responsive to radiotherapy. Metastatic disease is treated with platinum based chemotherapy.

QUESTION 42

A. TRUE   B. TRUE   C. FALSE   D. FALSE   E. TRUE

Hypercalcaemia can occur as a result of lytic bone lesions, include metastases from breast. Multiple myeloma is characterised by multiple bony deposits. Tertiary hyperparthyroidism may occur as aresult of prolonged renal failure.

QUESTION 43

A. TRUE   B. TRUE   C. TRUE   D. TRUE   E. TRUE

A wide range of clinical signs and symptoms may arise due to the metabolic stimulation of excessive thyroid hormone activity.

QUESTION 44

A. TRUE   B. TRUE   C. TRUE   D. FALSE   E. FALSE

Zollinger–Ellison syndrome involves the presence of fulminant peptic ulceration due to excessive gastrin production resulting in hyperacidity. The most common cause is due to G-cell tumours of the pancreatic islet cells, an this can be in association with MEN I syndrome. Raised serum gastrin is diagnostic.

QUESTION 45

A. TRUE   B. FALSE   C. TRUE   D. TRUE   E. FALSE

The female breast is a modified sweat gland, formed from the invagination of ectodermal cells into the underlying mesenchyme. The milk lines run from axilla to groin. Approximately 25% of the lymph drainage of the breast occurs through nodes other than the ipsilateral axilla.

QUESTION 46

A. FALSE   B. TRUE   C. FALSE   D. FALSE   E. TRUE

T4 is any form of advanced disease. Paget's disease is classed as TIS. Internal mammary node involvement is N3.

QUESTION 47

A. FALSE   B. FALSE   C. FALSE   D. FALSE   E. FALSE

Male breast cancer accounts for approximately 1% of all breast cancer cases. It is rare in younger men, the risk factors are unclear, but strong family history and exposure to carcinogens are included. Management of the lesion is the same as for the female variety.

QUESTION 48

A. TRUE   B. TRUE   C. FALSE   D. TRUE   E. TRUE

All cases need further investigation. Unconjugated neonatal jaundice is normally physiological and resolves spontaneously.

QUESTION 49

A. TRUE   B. FALSE   C. TRUE   D. TRUE   E. FALSE

Other medical conditions include urinary tract infection, gastroenteritis and diabetes mellitus.

QUESTION 50

A. FALSE   B. TRUE   C. FALSE   D. TRUE   E. FALSE

Circumcision is most commonly carried out for religious or cultural reasons in the interests of hygiene. The medical indications are of severe balanitis due to a tight foreskin (phimosis). The foreskin is normally non-retractile in the neonate. Congenital penile abnormalities are a contraindication to circumcision as the foreskin is commonly used in reconstruction.

Exam 2

QUESTION 1

Increased risk of development of deep vein thrombosis (DVT) include

A. Dehydration
B. Pelvic Surgery
C. Aspirin
D. Malignancy
E. Excess Protein C production

QUESTION 2

Hyperkalaemia

A. Occurs in renal failure
B. Causes tented T waves on a 12 lead ECG
C. Is associated with metabolic alkalosis
D. Occurs after prolonged vomiting
E. May be treated with a dextrose/insulin infusion

QUESTION 3

Patients on long term oral steroids undergoing surgery

A. Should have pre-operative gastroscopy to exclude ulcers
B. Have a risk of post-operative Addisonian crisis
C. Require pre-operative dextrose or glucose infusions
D. Should not be given a pre-medication
E. Oral dose should be converted to intravenous equivalent during the peri-operative period

QUESTION 4

Dextrose-Saline solution

A. Consists of 0.9% saline and 5% glucose
B. Contains bicarbonate ions
C. Has an approximate osmolality of 300mOsmol/kg
D. Three litres in 24 hours infused is sufficient to maintain electrolyte balance
E. Has a pH of approximately 7

QUESTION 5

Thiopentone

- **A.** Is metabolised in the liver
- **B.** Causes necrosis of tissues if extravasation occurs
- **C.** Causes arterial vasoconstriction
- **D.** Is a non depolarising muscle relaxant
- **E.** Is a benzodiazapine like drug

QUESTION 6

Dead space in the respiratory tract ventilation

- **A.** Includes the trachea
- **B.** Is increased in ARDS
- **C.** Is increased in pulmonary embolism
- **D.** Can be reduced by increased ventilatory rate
- **E.** Is proportional to arterial oxygen concentration

QUESTION 7

Colloid solutions such as "Gelofusine", "Haemaccel" and "Hespan"

- **A.** Contain no sodium or potassium
- **B.** Consist of protein molecules which remain in the intravascular compartment
- **C.** May give rise to allergic reactions
- **D.** May cause a coagulopathy
- **E.** Should not be given in septicaemic shock

QUESTION 8

Causes of post-operative confusion may include

- **A.** Urinary tract infection
- **B.** Hypoxia
- **C.** Electrolyte imbalance
- **D.** Alcohol withdrawal
- **E.** Opiate overdose

QUESTION 9

Causes of post-operative pyrexia include

- **A.** Transfusion reaction
- **B.** Pseudomembranous colitis
- **C.** Pulmonary embolism
- **D.** Tissue trauma
- **E.** Thrombophlebitis

QUESTION 10

Features of the systemic inflammatory response syndrome (SIRS) include

- A. Core temperature <35°C
- B. Respiratory rate > 16/min
- C. Hypercapnia with PCO_2 > 6 kPa
- D. Tachycardia > 90bpm
- E. Metabolic alkalosis

QUESTION 11

HIV (human immunodeficiency virus)

- A. Has a higher incidence amongst homosexual men in the UK
- B. Has a 10% chance of being transmitted through needlestick injury
- C. Takes less than two weeks to produce antibody response
- D. Is not infective until after 10-12 weeks incubation
- E. Can pass in-utero to the fetus

QUESTION 12

Prolene (polypropylene) sutures

- A. Are absorbable
- B. Are monofilament
- C. Are braided
- D. Are suitable for vascular anastamosis
- E. Are not recommended for skin closure

QUESTION 13

Contraindications to laparoscopic abdominal surgery include

- A. Extensive abdominal scars
- B. Previous myocardial infarction
- C. Severe Chronic Obstructive Airways Disease
- D. Bladder outflow obstruction
- E. Intestinal Obstruction

QUESTION 14

During a routine appendicectomy

- A. An incision is made over McBurney's point, two-thirds the distance from the umbilicus to the anterior superior iliac spine
- B. The inferior epigastric artery is ligated
- C. The appendicular artery is diathermied
- D. The appendix base is crushed, tied and may be buried
- E. Mesenteric lymph nodes should be biopsied if seen

QUESTION 15

Indications for a CT scan following a head injury include

A. Post traumatic amnesia
B. CSF rhinhorrea
C. Persistant vomiting
D. Post-traumatic seizure
E. Deteriorating level of consciousness

QUESTION 16

Class III hypovolaemic shock is characterised by

A. Represents 30-40% blood volume loss
B. Bradycardia
C. Peripheral vasodilation
D. A drop in supine blood pressure
E. Confusion or agitation

QUESTION 17

The following serum biochemical markers are associated with the following malignancies

A. Alpha-feto-protein (AFP) and cholangiocarcinoma
B. Carcinoembryonic antigen (CEA) and rectal cancer
C. Human chorionic gonadotrophin (HCG) and malignant melanoma
D. CA 153 and prostate cancer
E. CA 125 and ovarian cancer

QUESTION 18

Human DNA

A. Consists of a deoxyribose double nucleus backbone
B. Consist of opposing purine and pyramidine nucleotides
C. Four base codons signify the making of a specific amino acid
D. Cytosine always opposes guanine
E. Only the "intron" portion of the molecule actually codes

QUESTION 19

The following conditions may predispose malignant transformation

A. Ulcerative colitis
B. Barrett's oesophagus
C. Familial adenomatous polyposis
D. Crohn's disease
E. Coeliac disease

QUESTION 20

Frequent complications following splenectomy can include

A. Deep vein thrombosis
B. Right lower lobe atelectasis
C. Streptococcal sepsis
D. Petechial rashes
E. Unexplained fevers

QUESTION 21

The following conditions occur due to the presence of circulating anti-bodies

A. Graves disease
B. Hashimoto thyroiditis
C. Reidel's thyroiditis
D. Myasthenia gravis
E. Motor neurone disease

QUESTION 22

Non-Hodgkin's Lymphoma (NHL)

A. Is characterised by Reed-Sternberg cells on lymph node biopsy
B. Arises only from the T-cell lymphocyte population
C. High grade lymphoma has a better prognosis than low grade
D. Classically present with night sweats
E. Includes Burkitt's lymphoma as a subtype

QUESTION 23

Complications of a CVP line insertion include

A. Tension pneumothorax
B. Air embolism
C. Arterial injury
D. Mediastinitis
E. Venous thrombosis

QUESTION 24

The following drugs have the associated side effects

A. Voltarol and peptic ulceration
B. Codeine and hepatitis
C. Spironolactone and hypokalaemia
D. Digoxin and gynaecomastia
E. Amiodarone and epididymitis

QUESTION 25

Subarachnoid haemorrhage (SAH)

A. Is diagnosed by the presence or many red cells in the CSF on lumbar puncture
B. Is due to a rupture of a middle meningeal artery aneurysm
C. May cause an obstructive hydrocephalus
D. Is treated with plasma heamodilution
E. May be complicated with cardiac arrythmias

QUESTION 26

An acoustic neuromma

A. Is a tumour of the Schwann cell sheath
B. Projects into the cerebellopontine angle, and can compress the 5th and 7th nerves
C. May present with contralateral deafness
D. Can cause symptoms of raised intracranial pressure due to distortion and compression of the 4th ventricle
E. Can be treated with localised radiotherapy

QUESTION 27

Complications of head and neck radiotherapy for cancer include

A. Cataract formation
B. Osteonecrosis of the maxilla
C. Otitis media
D. Encephalopathy
E. Tenesmus

QUESTION 28

Pancoast tumours

A. Are lung carcinoma arising in or around the hilum
B. Cause a unilateral, dilated pupil
C. Are rarely malignant
D. May present with ptosis
E. Erosion of ribs may be noted on the plain chest X-ray

QUESTION 29

Tetralogy of Fallot

A. Is the most common congenital heart defect
B. Presents with central cyanosis and finger clubbing
C. There is stenosis of the pulmonary tract
D. There is left ventricular hypertrophy
E. Can be repaired by the Blalock shunt, an anastomosis between left subclavian artery and left pulmonary vein

QUESTION 30

Peripheral arterial blood flow is decreased in the following situations

A. Thrombocytopenia
B. Small bowel obstruction
C. Hyperfibrinoginaemia
D. Polycythemia
E. Lymphoma

QUESTION 31

Complications following aortic aneurysm surgery include

A. Mesenteric infarction
B. Spinal cord ischaemia
C. Renal failure
D. Splenic haematoma
E. Aortoduodenal fistula

QUESTION 32

Raynaud's disease

A. Is more common in women
B. Is rarely bilateral
C. Is associated with systemic sclerosis
D. Can be exacerbated by stress
E. May be treated with prostacylin if there is arisk of gangrene

QUESTION 33

Osteomyelitis

A. Staphylococcus aureus is the most common organism
B. Salmonella infection is associated with patients with sickle cell disease
C. Rarely occur as a result of haematologous spread from a distant source
D. Most foci develop in the diaphysis segment of long bones
E. ESR and CRP are raised in the acute phase

QUESTION 34

Paget's disease of bone

A. Commonly occurs below the age of 40 years
B. Consists of mixed sclerotic and lytic bony lesions
C. Plasma alkaline phosphatase is normal
D. There is increased urinary excretion of hydroxyproline
E. Pre-disposes to sarcoma formation

QUESTION 35

Dislocation of the shoulder joint

A. Anterior is more common than posterior
B. Is associated with damage to the axillary nerve
C. Is associated with a fracture of the posterior glenoid (bony Bankart lesion)
D. There may be a fracture of the posterior humeral head (Hill Sachs lesion)
E. Repeated dislocation may result in avascular necrosis of the humeral head

QUESTION 36

Crohns' disease

A. Usually spares the anus
B. Is radiologically characterised by skip lesions and pseudopolyps
C. Transmural inflammation and giant cells are present on histology
D. May be complicated by toxic megacolon
E. Rarely becomes malignant

QUESTION 37

Chronic gastric ulcers

A. Are associated with gastric hyperacidity
B. Is associated with smoking
C. Is more common in men
D. Undergo malignant transformation in over 40% of cases
E. Pain is often relieved by eating light meals

QUESTION 38

Colo-rectal carcinoma

A. Is more common in men
B. Invariably occurs in patients with familial adenomatous polyposis (FAP)
C. Commonly spreads via lymph nodes to the inguinal region
D. Dukes stage B indicates the tumour is still confined to the bowel wall
E. Risk is increased in patients with ulcerative colitis

QUESTION 39

Carcinoma of the prostate

A. Rarely presents with metastases
B. Has a higher and has a worse prognosis in Afro-Caribbeans
C. Posterior invasion is deflected by the fascia of Denonvilliers
D. In the TNM classification, T3 indicated a fixed lesion
E. Metastatic disease is treated with anti-oestrogenic drugs

QUESTION 40

The ureter

A. Is longer in males than females
B. The course is retroperitoneal and medial to the tips of the lumbar spine transverse processes
C. Passes under the junction of the common iliac artery
D. If duplex and do not join along their course, the upper ureter at the renal pelvis inserts below and medial to its partner in the bladder
E. The pelvi-ureteric junction is a common site for obstruction

QUESTION 41

Causes of an acutely tender testicle include

A. Torsion of hydatid of Morgani
B. Mumps
C. Measles
D. Hydrocele
E. Varicocoele

QUESTION 42

The thyroid gland

A. Is derived from the 1st and 2nd pharyngeal pouches
B. Is supplied by the inferior thyroid arteries which arises from the external carotid artery
C. Contains cells of neural crest origin
D. Stores T3 and T4 bound to thyroxine-binding globulin (TBG)
E. Lies over the 4th–6th tracheal rings

QUESTION 43

Parathyroid hormone (PTH)

A. Is secreted by the parafollicular cells within the parathyroid gland
B. Is a steroid analogue
C. Increases phosphate excretion in the urine
D. Enhances the absorption of vitamin D from the gut
E. Stimulates osteoclastic activity

QUESTION 44

Multiple endocrine neoplasia syndromes

A. Result from abnormalities of the APUD (amine precursor uptake decarboxylase) cells
B. Type I includes carcinoma of the parathyroid gland
C. Are familial
D. Type II includes medullary carcinoma of the thyroid
E. Pituitary tumours may be present in type I syndromes

QUESTION 45

Breast cancer risks include

- **A.** Late menarche
- **B.** Late first pregnancy
- **C.** Late menopause
- **D.** Multiple sexual partners
- **E.** Prolonged oral contraceptive pill

QUESTION 46

During axillary dissection

- **A.** A level I clearance removes all nodes above the level of pectoralis minor
- **B.** The axillary vein marks the distal limit of dissection
- **C.** Damage to the intercostobrachial nerves results in sensory loss over the medial aspect of the upper arm
- **D.** The long thoracic nerve is usually sacrificed
- **E.** The thoracodorsal trunk lies anterio-laterally

QUESTION 47

The breast screening programme in the UK

- **A.** Invites women aged 50-64 years for initial screening
- **B.** Follow up screening is every 5 years
- **C.** Mammography and ultrasound is carried out on both breasts
- **D.** Abnormalities on the initial screen are biopsied
- **E.** The aim of the programme is to reduce deaths from breast cancer significantly

QUESTION 48

Infantile hypertrophic pyloric stenosis

- **A.** Is more common in male than female babies
- **B.** Is more common in the Afro-Caribbean population
- **C.** Presents with projectile, bilious vomiting
- **D.** Biochemical changes include low serum chloride, potassium and bicarbonate
- **E.** It is surgically treated with cutting of the pylorus muscle

QUESTION 49

Intussussception of bowel in children

- **A.** Occurs most commonly at 18 months
- **B.** Is more common in males
- **C.** Is associated with henoch-Schonlein purpura
- **D.** Is often characterised by a fullness in the right iliac fossa
- **E.** Reduction is perfomed with a flexible sigmoidoscope

QUESTION 50

Pelviureteric junction obstruction

A. Results in hydronephrosis without hydroureter
B. Is more common in males
C. May present with haematuria
D. Is usually associated with duplex ureters
E. May result in nephrectomy if the kidney is providing less than 10% of overall renal function

Exam 2: Answers

QUESTION 1

A. TRUE   B. TRUE   C. FALSE   D. TRUE   E. FALSE

Deep vein thrombosis is precipitated by any factors increasing the viscosity or level of stasis of blood within the veins. Prolonged surgery, in particular abdominal, pelvic, orthopaedic and that for malignant disease increase risk. Aspirin reduces platelet aggregation, and protein C, S or anti-thrombin III deficiency increase coagulability.

QUESTION 2

A. TRUE   B. TRUE   C. FALSE   D. FALSE   E. TRUE

Hyperkalaemia changes occurs in the presence of a serum $K^+ > 6.0$ mmol/l. It appears in chronic renal failure and acutely in diabetic ketoacidosis. Potassium is lost in vomiting and diarrhea. Calcium gluconate, or dextrose /insulin infusions temporarily reduce hyperkalaemia.

QUESTION 3

A. FALSE   B. TRUE   C. FALSE   D. FALSE   E. TRUE

Patients on long term steroids may have adrenal suppression with a risk of post-operative Addisonian crisis. The peri-operative period should be covered with intravenous hydrocortisone until normal oral intake is re-established.

QUESTION 4

A. FALSE   B. FALSE   C. TRUE   D. FALSE   E. FALSE

Dextrose-Saline solution is 0.18% NaCl, 4% glucose, contains 31 mmol/l of sodium and chorine ions, has an osmolality of 284 mOsmol/kg and a pH of 4.5. Additional potassium is required to fulfil electrolyte balance.

QUESTION 5

A. TRUE   B. TRUE   C. TRUE   D. FALSE   E. FALSE

Thiopentone is a sulphur containing barbiturate, intravenous anaesthetic agent. It causes tissue necrosis if extravasated, and may cause peripheral ischemia if injected into an artery.

QUESTION 6

A. TRUE   B. TRUE   C. TRUE   D. FALSE   E. FALSE

Dead space consists of area which are ventilated but not perfused (anatomical) and those which are perfused but not ventilated. Under ventilation of alveoli will cause a rise in arterial pCO_2.

QUESTION 7

A. FALSE   B. FALSE   C. TRUE   D. TRUE   E. FALSE

The colloid solutions named consist of large molecules derived from gelatin in the case of gelofusine and haemaccel, and starch in the case of Hespan. They are useful in temporarily maintaining the intravascular volume in emergency situations.

QUESTION 8

A. TRUE   B. TRUE   C. TRUE   D. TRUE   E. FALSE

All causes are more common in the elderly or in those with pre-existing dementia or psychiatric conditions. Opiate overdose causes drowsiness.

QUESTION 9

A. TRUE   B. TRUE   C. TRUE   D. TRUE   E. TRUE

Post-operative pyrexia can be infectious or non-infectious. The latter include surgical tissue damage, drug reaction, pulmonary atelectasis.

QUESTION 10

A. TRUE   B. FALSE   C. FALSE   D. TRUE   E. FALSE

Sepsis is defined as the development of a systemic inflammatory response syndrome. This may cause progression to multi-organ dysfunction syndrome.

QUESTION 11

A. TRUE   B. FALSE   C. FALSE   D. FALSE   E. TRUE

HIV has a 0.4% chance of being transmitted following needlestick injury. It take 6–12 weeks to produce a detectable antibody response but is infective in this period.

QUESTION 12

A. FALSE   B. TRUE   C. FALSE   D. TRUE   E. FALSE

Prolene is a nonabsorbable synthetic suture.

QUESTION 13

A. TRUE   B. FALSE   C. FALSE   D. FALSE   E. TRUE

Risks of laparoscopic surgery increase with intra-abdominal adhesions or distended viscera. Pneumoperitoneum interferes with respiratory function.

QUESTION   14

A. TRUE   B. FALSE   C. FALSE   D. TRUE   E. FALSE

A transverse Lanz or an oblique Gridiron incision is usually used. The inferior epigastric vessels are not usually seen in the approaches. The vessels supplying the appendix should be tied. Mesenteric lymph nodes are not routinely biopsied unless there is a suspicion of malignancy or TB.

QUESTION   15

A. FALSE   B. TRUE   C. FALSE   D. TRUE   E. TRUE

Any suspicion of an intracranial bleed should have a low threshold for scanning.

QUESTION   16

A. TRUE   B. FALSE   C. FALSE   D. TRUE   E. TRUE

Haemorrhage of 1500-2000 mls in an adult represents severe blood loss. There is tachycardia, tachypneoa, falling arterial pressure and tissue hypoxia.

QUESTION   17

A. FALSE   B. TRUE   C. FALSE   D. FALSE   E. TRUE

"Tumour markers" are generally unreliable in the primary diagnosis or in screening for common malignancies. They do however have a role in monitoring some diseases. A negatively raised marker therefore does not exclude presence of the associated malignancy.

PSA and Ca125 are raised in prostatic and ovarian cancer respectively. CEA is raised in all malignancies of the GI tract, but more frequently in colorectal cancer. HCG is raised in pregnancy and in trophoblastic tumours. AFP is raised in hepatocellular carcinoma and testicular and ovarian teratoma. Ca153 is associated with breast cancer.

QUESTION   18

A. TRUE   B. TRUE   C. FALSE   D. TRUE   E. FALSE

Sequences of three codons signify a specific amino acid. Only exons are expressed.

QUESTION   19

A. TRUE   B. TRUE   C. TRUE   D. FALSE   E. TRUE

Lesion in FAP invariably become malignant. UC, Barrett's, and Coeliac disease have a 10 -15% chance of transformation. Lesions in Crohn's disease are not regarded as pre-malignant.

QUESTION   20

A. TRUE   B. FALSE   C. TRUE   D. FALSE   E. TRUE

There is thrombocytosis following splenectomy and increased susceptibility to infections from Streptococcal, Meningococcus and Haemophilus bacteria. Fever may also occur without explanation.

QUESTION 21

A. TRUE   B. TRUE   C. FALSE   D. TRUE   E. FALSE

Reidel's thyroiditis is probably viral in origin. In myasthenia there are circulating antibodies against acetylcholine receptors at the neuromuscular junction. The aetiology of motor neurone disease is not clear.

QUESTION 22

A. FALSE   B. FALSE   C. TRUE   D. FALSE   E. TRUE

Various subtypes of lymphoma are classified as NHL, are divided into high and low grade, and can arise from B and T cells. Most patients present with lymph node enlargement without systemic symptoms.

QUESTION 23

A. FALSE   B. TRUE   C. TRUE   D. FALSE   E. TRUE

Tension pneumothorax requires a one way valve mechanism which is unlikely with simple line insertion.

QUESTION 24

A. TRUE   B. FALSE   C. FALSE   D. TRUE   E. TRUE

Spironolactone retains potassium at the expense of sodium and water.

QUESTION 25

A. FALSE   B. FALSE   C. TRUE   D. TRUE   E. TRUE

Spontaneous SAH is most commonly due to a ruptured congenital aneurysm of the circle of Willis. Xanthochromia in the lumbar puncture CSF in addition to a clinical picture is diagnostic.

QUESTION 26

A. TRUE   B. TRUE   C. FALSE   D. TRUE   E. FALSE

Growth of an acoustic neuroma normally impinges on the 5th and 7th nerves causing symptoms including trigeminal neuralgia and facial weakness.

QUESTION 27

A. TRUE   B. TRUE   C. TRUE   D. TRUE   E. FALSE

All complications are more likely to occur if re-radiation becomes necessary. In addition cranial nerves may become affected.

QUESTION 28

A. FALSE   B. FALSE   C. FALSE   D. TRUE   E. TRUE

Pancost tumours are lung carcinoma arising at the apex. Invasion of the ribs, lower brachial plexus and sympathetic chain can give rise to a Horner's syndrome including unilateral ptosis and pupillary constriction.

QUESTION 29

A. TRUE   B. TRUE   C. TRUE   D. FALSE   E. FALSE

Fallot's tetralogy accounts for 10% of congenital heart defects, and is the most common. Variable degrees of central cyanosis are noted. The defect consist of pulmonary tract stenosis, ventricular septal defect, overriding aorta, and right ventricular hypertrophy. Blalock shunt anastamoses the left subclavian and left pulmonary arteries.

QUESTION 30

A. FALSE   B. TRUE   C. TRUE   D. TRUE   E. FALSE

Arterial blood flow is inversely related to viscosity, which increases with a raised heamatocrit.

QUESTION 31

A. TRUE   B. TRUE   C. TRUE   D. FALSE   E. TRUE

Damage to all vascular structures arising from the aorta may occur. Aorto–duodenal fistula is a late complication.

QUESTION 32

A. TRUE   B. FALSE   C. TRUE   D. TRUE   E. TRUE

Raynaud's disease is a vasospastic condition occuring bilaterally. It is more common in women and associated with smoking and some auto–immune conditions. Sympathectomy is successful in 30-40% of cases.

QUESTION 33

A. TRUE   B. TRUE   C. FALSE   D. FALSE   E. TRUE

Most infections occur as a result of haematologus spread from a distal source, and tend to locate at the epiphyseal and metaphyseal regions of the long bones.

QUESTION 34

A. FALSE   B. TRUE   C. FALSE   D. TRUE   E. TRUE

The aetiology of Paget's disease is unknown, but the incidence increases with age, and is rare below 50. There is raised serum alkaline phosphatase and urinary hydroxyproline.

QUESTION 35

A. TRUE   B. TRUE   C. FALSE   D. TRUE   E. FALSE

Posterior dislocation is rare and is documented as following epileptic seizures or electrocution. The brachial plexus and axillary nerve are at risk in a dislocation. The Bankart lesion consists of damage to the anteror glenoid. Recurrent dislocation requires investigation and surgical correction of any associated lesions.

QUESTION 36

A. FALSE B. FALSE C. FALSE D. FALSE E. FALSE

Crohn's disease can affect any and multiple points in the GI tract, and consists of a transmural inflammatory process with granuloma present. Pseudopolyps, toxic megacolon and malignant change are related to ulcerative colitis.

QUESTION 37

A. FALSE B. TRUE C. FALSE D. FALSE E. FALSE

Chronic gastric ulcers are associated with normal or acid hyposecretion, or atrophic gastritis. It is less common than duodenal ulceration, and the incidence in men and women is about equal. Some gastric ulcers become malignant, but the incidence is less than 5%. Typically, pain associated with gastric ulcers occurs soon after eating, and the patient may develop a fear of eating and hence weight loss.

QUESTION 38

A. TRUE B. TRUE C. FALSE D. FALSE E. TRUE

Colorectal cancer is the second most common malignancy in the UK it is more common in men. Pre-existing lesions and familial predisposition are risk factors. Lymph node spread is common, but this tends to be upward and lateral. Dukes B stage indicates complete penetration of the bowel wall.

QUESTION 39

A. FALSE B. TRUE C. TRUE D. FALSE E. FALSE

Prostatic cancer occurs most commonly after 65 years and has a higher incidence in Afro-Caribbeans and less in the Oriental population. Posterior tumours tend to be deflected upwards and may block the ureteral orifices. Stage T3 indicates extension outside the capsule, T4 indicates a fixed lesion. Hormonal manipulation is using testosterone suppressing agents.

QUESTION 40

A. FALSE B. FALSE C. FALSE D. TRUE E. TRUE

The ureter is 25 cm long in both sexes in the adult. It is retroperitoneal in the upper half and enters the pelvis in the lower half, passing over the bifurcation of the common iliac artery, and lateral to the transverse processes.

QUESTION 41

A. TRUE B. TRUE C. FALSE D. FALSE E. FALSE

Torsion of the testicle must be excluded in all cases of an acutely tender testicle. Mumps can cause orchitis, and infections of the epididymis can also give rise to testicular pain. Hydroceles and Varicocoeles cause swelling but rarely pain.

QUESTION 42

A. TRUE   B. FALSE   C. TRUE   D. FALSE   E. FALSE

The thyroid gland develops from ectoderm of the 1st and 2nd pharyngeal pouches, and also receives cells from the ultimo-branchial body of the 4th pouch which originate from the neural crest and become the parafollicular or C-cells. T3 and T4 are bound to thyroglobulin in the thyroid and to TBG and TBPA in the plasma.

QUESTION 43

A. FALSE   B. FALSE   C. TRUE   D. FALSE   E. TRUE

PTH is secreted by the chief and oxyphil cells of the parathyroid gland. It is a 84 amino acid polypeptide, whose overall activity is to increase serum calcium and reduce calcium phosphate. Vitamin D (cholecalciferol) is synthesised in the skin under the influence of ultraviolet light. This undergoes hydroxylation first in the liver, then the kidney. The second stage is increased by PTH. The effect of the hydoxylated vitamin D is to increase calcium and phosphate absorption from the gut.

QUESTION 44

A. TRUE   B. FALSE   C. TRUE   D. TRUE   E. TRUE

MEN I consists of parathyroid hyperplasia, pancreatic endocrine tumours, and tumours of the anterior pituitary. MEN II consists of parathyroid hyperplasia, medullary carcinoma of the thyroid and phaechromocytoma.

QUESTION 45

A. FALSE   B. TRUE   C. TRUE   D. FALSE   E. TRUE

Prolonged or uninterrupted exposure to any oestrogenic stimulus is a risk factor.

QUESTION 46

A. FALSE   B. TRUE   C. TRUE   D. FALSE   E. FALSE

Axillary clearance (Level III) removes all nodes below the axillary vein. A Level I clearance limits the dissection to below the pectoralis minor. The intercostobrachial nerve is often damaged during dissection, but the long thoracic, situated on the medial wall, supplying serratus anterior, and the thoracodorsal trunk which lies posteriorly in the axilla must be identified and preserved.

QUESTION 47

A. TRUE   B. FALSE   C. FALSE   D. FALSE   E. TRUE

Screening initially involves two views on a mammogram, and if this is normal, recalls are after 3 years. If abnormalities are detected, then routine assessment is carried out in a breast unit. The results of the programme are still under evaluation.

QUESTION 48

A. TRUE   B. FALSE   C. FALSE   D. FALSE   E. FALSE

Pyloric stenosis occurs more commonly in males with a ratio of 4:1. It is more common in Europeans. Vomiting is of feed, not bilious, and serum bicarbonate levels rise. A Ramstedt's pyloromyotomy involves splitting of the muscle layers.

QUESTION 49

A. FALSE   B. TRUE   C. TRUE   D. FALSE   E. FALSE

The common age of presentation is between 5 and 9 months, and is slightly more common in males. It is associated with Meckel's, lymphoid hyperplasia, lymphomas and any other mucosal lesions, including haematoma which may occur in Henoch–Schönlein purpura.

There is an emptiness in the right iliac fossa (Dance's sign) and a mass palpable in the right hypochondrium. Reduction and diagnosis is done in the first instance under hydrostatic pressure via a Barium enema.

QUESTION 50

A. TRUE   B. TRUE   C. TRUE   D. FALSE   E. TRUE

This is a congenital abnormality associated with disorganised tissue. It is diagnosed using ultrasound, and renal function then needs to be assessed. If kidney function is satisfactory, and the patient symptomatic then a pyeloplasty may be carried out.

Exam 3

QUESTION 1

Deranged clotting function commonly occurs in patients with

A. Malnutrition
B. Cirrhosis
C. Hypothyroidism
D. Protein C deficiency
E. Insulin dependent diabetes mellitus

QUESTION 2

Hypertension

A. Is a contraindication to surgery if the diastolic blood pressure exceeds 115 mmHg
B. Occurs in Conn's syndrome
C. If uncontrolled, increases the risk of post-operative bleeding
D. May cause left ventricular hypertrophy
E. Is exacerbated in suboptimal post-operative analgesia

QUESTION 3

The oral contraceptive pill

A. Progestrone-only type is not usually associated with surgical problems
B. The combination oestrogen-progestrone pill is associated with increased post-operative bleeding
C. Is usually stopped six months prior to elective surgery
D. Should be augmented with other forms of contraception post-operatively
E. Surgical risks are potentiated in smokers

QUESTION 4

Muscle relaxation during surgery

A. Allows improved intra-abdominal access
B. Is not necessary in ventilated patients
C. Is maintained using a depolarising agent such as suxamethonium
D. Block acetyl-choline receptors on muscle end plates
E. Side effects include histamine release

QUESTION   5

Myocardial function may be significantly affected by the following

A. Halothane
B. Thiopentone
C. Suxamethonium
D. Metoclopromide
E. Fentanyl

QUESTION   6

The binding of haemoglobin to oxygen

A. Follows a linear relationship
B. Is over 90% saturated when the partial pressure of oxygen is 10 kPa
C. Is approximately 70% saturated in venous blood
D. Is increased with increased pH
E. Is increased in sickle cell disease

QUESTION   7

Pulmonary oedema is characterised by

A. Diminshed air entry in the lung bases
B. Dyspneoa
C. Respiratory acidosis
D. Kerley B lines
E. Hypercapnia

QUESTION   8

The following infections can be transmitted through blood transfusion

A. Human Immundeficiency Virus
B. Cytomegalovirus
C. Malaria
D. Hepatitis C
E. Clostridium difficile

QUESTION   9

Post-operative cholecystitis

A. Only occurs in the presence of gallstones
B. Commonly causes jaundice
C. Can be diagnosed with a CT scan
D. May cause mucosal ischaemia and perforation
E. Surgery is contraindicated

QUESTION 10

Prophylactic antibiotics are routinely administered in the following procedures

A. Total hip replacement
B. Endoscopic biliary stent for obstructive jaundice
C. Mastectomy
D. Mesh hernia repair
E. Colonoscopy

QUESTION 11

Factors which increase the risk of pneumonia developing in surgical patients include

A. Prolonged ventilation with endo tracheal tube
B. Increased gastric motility
C. Oesophago-gastric incompetence
D. Reduced salivary secretions
E. Increased gastric acidity

QUESTION 12

Lignocaine

A. Blocks type C nerve fibres first
B. Should not be used in ring blocks for fingers
C. Has a long half life
D. The maximal dose increases if adrenaline is added
E. Should not be used in epidural anaesthesia

QUESTION 13

Factors which reduce the likelihood of anastomotic leak following a small bowel resection include

A. Using non-absorbable sutures
B. Placing the bowel ends under moderate tension
C. Naso-gastric decompression of the bowel if obstructed
D. Oversewing the mesentery
E. Using a second suture layer to evert the serosa

QUESTION 14

Safety precautions for operating on high risk patients should include

A. Double gloving
B. Protective goggles
C. Waterproof disposable gowns
D. Blunt needles
E. Maximal numbers of operating and theatre staff involved

QUESTION   15

Indications for urgent laparotomy following trauma include

- **A.** Penetrating knife injuries
- **B.** Splenic haematoma
- **C.** Pelvic fracture
- **D.** Frank haematuria
- **E.** Raised amylase

QUESTION   16

Urethral damage following general trauma

- **A.** Is often an isolated injury
- **B.** Often follows straddling injuries
- **C.** If blood is seen at the urethral meatus urethral catheterisation should not be attempted
- **D.** Can be assessed with an IVU
- **E.** Long term complications include stricture formation

QUESTION   17

The following tumours can show good responses to conventional systemic chemotherapy

- **A.** Malignant melanoma
- **B.** Wilm's tumour
- **C.** Breast cancer
- **D.** Acute lymphoblastic leukaemia
- **E.** Pancreatic cancer

QUESTION   18

The following conditions are associated with mutations of a tumour suppression genes

- **A.** Retinoblastoma
- **B.** Polyposis coli
- **C.** Barrets oesopahgus
- **D.** Wilms tumour
- **E.** Cervical Intraepithelial neoplasia

QUESTION   19

The syndromes listed are associated with the following tumours

- **A.** Von Hippel–Lindau and renal cell carcinoma
- **B.** Neurofibromatosis and phaechromocytoma
- **C.** Tyrosinaemia and pancreatic cancer
- **D.** Albinism and basal cell carcinoma
- **E.** Peutz – Jegher's and colorectal carcinoma

QUESTION 20

Indications for splenectomy include

A. Malaria
B. Idiopathic thrombocytopenic purpura (ITP)
C. Hereditory sphercytosis
D. Sarcoidosis
E. Budd-Chiari syndrome

QUESTION 21

Disseminated intravascular coagulation (DIC)

A. May follow severe trauma
B. Results in a hypercoagulable state
C. Results in the widespread deposition of fibrin in small vessels
D. May precipitate fat embolism
E. Should be treated with intravenous steroids

QUESTION 22

Leukaemia

A. Acute lymphoblastic leukaemia is a disease of childhood
B. The Philadelphia chromosome is associated with chronic myeloid leukaemia
C. Acute myeloid leukaemia usually follows infection with the HTLV-1 virus
D. Splenomegaly is most commonly associated with chronic myeloid leukaemia
E. Chronic lymphocytic leukaemia is most commonly a proliferation of B-cells

QUESTION 23

A chest drain for a left sided pneumothorax

A. Should be connected via an underwater seal
B. Should be aimed toward the apex
C. Should be inserted in the second intercostal space, mid-clavicular line
D. Is positioned under general anaesthetic
E. Is introduced on a trocar

QUESTION 24

The following drugs are not recommeded during pregnancy

A. Warfarin
B. Folic acid
C. Paracetamol
D. Lithium
E. Sodium valproate

QUESTION 25

The fifth cranial nerve (trigeminal)

A. Consist of three divisions which contain mixed motor and sensory fibres
B. Is the largest cranial nerve
C. The first division (ophthalamic) splits into three branches all which leave the cranium via the superior orbital fissure
D. The second division (maxillary) is sensory to lower eyelid
E. The third division (mandibular) supplies the muscles of mastication except tensor palati and tensor tympani

QUESTION 26

Early symptoms and signs of rising intracranial pressure include

A. Headache, nausea and vomiting
B. Neck stiffness and photophobia
C. Pupillary dilatation
D. Bradycardia
E. Falling systolic blood pressure

QUESTION 27

The larynx

A. Is made up of three single and two paired cartliges
B. The false cords are found within the subglottic region
C. The internal branch of the superior laryngeal nerve provides a sensory mucosal innervation
D. The epiglottis lies outside the larynx
E. The recurrent laryngeal nerve supplies the cricothyroid muscle

QUESTION 28

Bronchial carcinoma

A. Common risk factors include asbestos exposure
B. Is the most common cancer in the UK
C. Adenocarcinoma is the most common subtype
D. Small cell tumours have the best prognosis
E. Can secrete steroid hormones

QUESTION 29

Mitral valve stenosis

A. When associated with rheumatic fever is more common in men
B. Causes hypertrophy of the left ventricle
C. Can precipitate mesenteric infarction
D. Clinically there is a pansystolic murmur
E. Infective endocarditis is a frequent complication

QUESTION   30

Risk factors for atherosclerosis include

A. Smoking
B. High plasma high density lipoprotein cholesterol
C. Hypofibrinogenaemia
D. High plasma factor VIIIc
E. Thrombocytosis

QUESTION   31

Venous gangrene

A. Can occur in the presence of normal arterial pulsation
B. Is associated with underlying visceral malignancy
C. Is associated with renal failure
D. Is associated with polycythemia rubra vera
E. Always involves the full depth of tissues

QUESTION   32

Graduated compression stockings in the treatment of chronic venous ulcers

A. Is contra-indicated in diabetics
B. Should allow a pressure of 30 mmHg at the ankle
C. The pressure should be high around the knee joint
D. Treatment should be used with diuretics
E. Standard bandaging consists of four layers

QUESTION   33

Gout

A. Is a disorder of pyramidine metabolism characterised by hyperuricaemia
B. Uric acid and calcium pyrophosphate crystals may be isolated from synovial fluid
C. Occurs more commonly in the small joints
D. Is treated with allopurinol in the acute phase
E. Is associated with renal failure

QUESTION   34

Osteomalacia

A. Is defined as decreased mineralisation of bone
B. Is characteristic of a "trefoil pelvis" and Looser's zone on plain pelvic X-ray
C. Is associated with hypercalcaemia
D. Is associated with chronic renal failure
E. Pre-disposes to sarcoma formation

QUESTION 35

Complications of fractures include

A. Myositis ossificans
B. Endarteritis obliterans
C. Volkmann's ischaemic contracture
D. Sudek's atrophy
E. Fat embolism

QUESTION 36

Femoral hernia

A. Are more common in men than women
B. Are more common than inguinal hernia in women
C. Are more common in nulliparous women
D. Emerge lateral to the Femoral vein
E. Carry a relatively high risk of strangulation

QUESTION 37

Acute duodenal perforation

A. Is more common in men than women, with highest incidence between 40- 60 years age group.
B. The lesion typically occurs on the posterior duodenal surface
C. Urgent diagnostic endoscopy is indicated
D. Air is present under the diaphragm on an erect plain chest X-ray in over 95% of cases
E. A characteristic "double bubble" sign is seen on supine abdominal X-rays

QUESTION 38

Raised gastrin levels can occur with

A. Pernicious anaemia
B. Gastric obstruction
C. Renal failure
D. MEN I syndrome
E. Zollinger-Ellison syndrome

QUESTION 39

Acute prostatitis

A. Can be bacterial, with common pathogens including E. Coli and Staph. aureus
B. Usually originates from a kidney infection and descends down
C. Can present with rigors
D. If complicated by an abscess requires drainage
E. Can be a complication heamorrhoidal injection

QUESTION 40

Causes of bilateral hydronephrosis include

A. Carcinoma of the cervix
B. Horseshoe kidney
C. Carcinoma of the rectum
D. Stricture of the urethral meatus
E. Carcinoma of the rectum

QUESTION 41

Following spinal trauma resulting in paraplegia

A. The bladder initially becomes distended
B. The bladder should be drained after injury
C. May be suitable to treatment with urinary diversion
D. Self catheterisation is rarely successful
E. Renal stone disease is a long term complication

QUESTION 42

Papillary carcinoma of the thyroid

A. Occurs commonly in geographically iodine depleted areas
B. Occurs mainly in elderly patients
C. Is frequently multi-focal
D. Spreads mainly to paratracheal and cervical lymph nodes lymph nodes
E. Is characterised histologically by the presence of "Orphan Annie" cells and psammoma bodies

QUESTION 43

Primary hyperparathyroidism

A. In most cases is due to carcinoma of the parathyroid
B. Is associated with multiple endocrine neoplasia syndromes (MEN)
C. May present with kidney stones
D. Can be diagnosed clinically through Chvostek's sign is severe cases
E. Can cause finger clubbing

QUESTION 44

Primary hyperaldosteronism (Conn's syndrome)

A. Results from a tumour within the adrenal medulla
B. There is increased circulating levels of angiotensin
C. Serum renin levels are high
D. There is a metabolic alkalosis
E. Can be initially treated medically with spironolactone

QUESTION 45

A bloody nipple discharge is commonly associated with

A. Duct ectasia
B. Intraductal papilloma
C. Fibrocystic disease
D. Prolactinoma
E. Mondor's disease

QUESTION 46

Gynaecomastia (swelling of the male breast) is

A. Most commonly due to an underlying breast malignancy
B. Often occurs in adolescent boys
C. May be caused by digoxin
D. Is associated with cirrhosis of the liver
E. Is reduced with steroid treatment

QUESTION 47

Tamoxifen in the adjuvant treatement of breast cancer

A. Side effects include hot flushes, loss of libido and vaginal dryness
B. There is a increased risk of thrombo-embolic disease
C. Use is contraindicated if the tumour is oestrogen receptor negative
D. The greatest benefit is seen in post-menopausal women
E. Unless side-effects are not tolerated, it should be taken for a minimum of two years

QUESTION 48

Wilms' tumour

A. May be associated with mental retardation
B. Is associated with the WT gene on chromosome 11
C. Most commonly presents between 5 and 10 years
D. Sarcomatous change is associated with poorer prognosis
E. Is locally invasive

QUESTION 49

Undescended testes

A. Occur in 1 in 10 000 boys
B. The most common location is in the femoral region
C. Is associated with normal fertility
D. Is associated with increased risk of malignancy
E. Orchidopexy is indicated at five years old

QUESTION   50

Inguinal hernia in children

A. Is more common in pre-term infants
B. Is associated with cryptorchidism
C. Is approximately equal in boys and girls
D. Should be repaired using a prolene mesh technique
E. The contralateral groin should be routinely explores to exclude bilateral hernia

Exam 3: Answers

QUESTION 1

A. TRUE   B. TRUE   C. FALSE   D. FALSE   E. FALSE

Deranged clotting is most commonly due to alteration of liver or platelet function. Malnutrition and cirrhosis diminish hepatic function.

QUESTION 2

A. TRUE   B. TRUE   C. TRUE   D. TRUE   E. TRUE

Previously undiagnosed hypertension may become apparent for the first time prior to surgery. If possible, surgery should be postponed until investigations are carried out and the blood pressure correctly regulated.

QUESTION 3

A. TRUE   B. FALSE   C. FALSE   D. TRUE   E. TRUE

The combination pill increases the risk of DVT in women undergoing surgery, particularly in smokers. It is usually stopped six weeks prior to elective surgery, and alternative contraception should be used to compensate for reduced absorption.

QUESTION 4

A. TRUE   B. FALSE   C. FALSE   D. TRUE   E. TRUE

Depolarisng agents (e.g. suxamethonium) are short acting. Non depolarising agents (e.g. atracurium, vecuronium, pancuronium) are longer lasting. Side-effects include histamine release, bradycardia and rarely hyperpyrexia.

QUESTION 5

A. TRUE   B. TRUE   C. TRUE   D. FALSE   E. FALSE

Fentanyl cause very slight myocardial contractility. This is considerably more significant with suxamethonium, thiopentone and halothane.

QUESTION 6

A. FALSE   B. TRUE   C. TRUE   D. TRUE   E. FALSE

The affinity of oxygen to haemoglobin follows a sigmoid relationship with almost complete satura-tion over a partial pressure of 10 kPa. In venous blood, with a pO_2 of approximately 5 kPa, the haemoglobin is still 70% saturated. Affinity for oxygen is decreased with raised H^+ concentration, temperature and levels of 2,3 DPG.

QUESTION 7

A. FALSE   B. TRUE   C. FALSE   D. TRUE   E. FALSE

Pulmonary oedema presents with dyspnoea and crepitations at the lung bases. There is hypoxia, and CO_2 is blown off causing a respiratory alkalosis.

QUESTION 8

A. TRUE   B. TRUE   C. TRUE   D. TRUE   E. FALSE

Clostridium difficile is normally a gut pathogen.

QUESTION 9

A. FALSE   B. FALSE   C. TRUE   D. TRUE   E. FALSE

A calculous cholecystits may occur following major surgery. Presentation may be with pain and a right upper quadrant mass and sepsis. Failure to resolve requires emergency decompression and or cholecystectomy.

QUESTION 10

A. TRUE   B. TRUE   C. FALSE   D. TRUE   E. FALSE

Any procedure involving an implant or prosthesis, or potentially releasing bacteria systemically will benefit from antibiotics.

QUESTION 11

A. TRUE   B. FALSE   C. TRUE   D. TRUE   E. FALSE

Decreased gastric acidity, motility, salivary secretions and oesophageal competence result in increased risk of bacterial colonisation and pneumonia on aspiration.

QUESTION 12

A. TRUE   B. FALSE   C. FALSE   D. TRUE   E. FALSE

Lignocaine is a short acting local anaesthetic which acts on small diameter pain fibres. Addition of adrenaline prevents use in the extremities but allows increased dosage.

QUESTION 13

A. FALSE   B. FALSE   C. TRUE   D. FALSE   E. FALSE

Anastomotic leak is unlikely if the bowel ends are viable, vascularised and not under tension. Care must be taken when closing the mesenteric defect not to compromise vascularity.

QUESTION 14

A. TRUE   B. TRUE   C. TRUE   D. TRUE   E. FALSE

High risk patients such as HIV should be operated on by the minimal number, but most experienced medical and nursing staff available. Universal precautions reduce the risk of incidental needlestick or splash accident.

QUESTION 15

A. TRUE   B. TRUE   C. FALSE   D. FALSE   E. FALSE

Splenic haematoma are unlikely to resolve on conservative management, unlike liver or kidney trauma.

QUESTION 16

A. FALSE   B. TRUE   C. FALSE   D. FALSE   E. FALSE

Damage to the various segments of the urethra rarely occur in isolation, and are often associated with major trama including pelvic fractures. Urethral catheterisation may be carefully attempted, and if this fails, suprapubic catheterisation. A urethrogram is the investigation of choice.

QUESTION 17

A. FALSE   B. TRUE   C. TRUE   D. TRUE   E. FALSE

Chemotherapy may be curative in some cases and used as adjuvant treatment in others.

QUESTION 18

A. TRUE   B. TRUE   C. FALSE   D. TRUE   E. FALSE

Rb, APC, and WT1 genes are associated with retinoblastoma, polyposis coli, and Wilms tumours respectively.

QUESTION 19

A. TRUE   B. TRUE   C. FALSE   D. TRUE   E. FALSE

Tyrosinaemia is linked with hepatocellular carcinoma. Peutz-Jeghers syndrome is linked with ovarian and small bowel malignancies.

QUESTION 20

A. FALSE   B. TRUE   C. TRUE   D. FALSE   E. FALSE

Other than trauma, splenectomy improves ITP if medical management has failed. The spleen may also be removed in extensive gastric cancer and pancreatic cancer surgery.

QUESTION   21

A. TRUE   B. FALSE   C. TRUE   D. FALSE   E. FALSE

DIC may occur as a result of trauma, sepsis or any other major systemic insult. There is activation of the clotting cascade at the expense of clotting factors, and deposition of fibrin. This results in cell lysis and a bleeding tendency.

QUESTION   22

A. TRUE   B. TRUE   C. FALSE   D. TRUE   E. TRUE

Leukaemia has a overall incidence of 5/100 000, and can be sub-divided into acute and chronic, and lymphoid or myeloid.

QUESTION   23

A. TRUE   B. TRUE   C. FALSE   D. FALSE   E. FALSE

A definitive chest drain for a pneumothorax is normally placed in the 5th intercostal space, mid-axillary line. It is normal to do this under local anaesthetic and the use of a trocar is not recommended.

QUESTION   24

A. TRUE   B. FALSE   C. FALSE   D. TRUE   E. TRUE

Anti-convulsants have a teratogenic effect, but this must be weighed against the risk of uncontrolled seizures

QUESTION   25

A. FALSE   B. TRUE   C. TRUE   D. TRUE   E. FALSE

Only the third division is mixed, the rest are sensory. All muscles of mastication are supplied by the mandibular branch.

QUESTION   26

A. TRUE   B. FALSE   C. FALSE   D. TRUE   E. FALSE

Neck stiffness and photophobia are signs of meningism, and pupillary dilatation occurs in third nerve palsy, all of which would be very late signs occurring prior to coning. Bradycardia and a rising blood pressure is known as the Cushing response to raised intracranial pressure.

QUESTION   27

A. FALSE   B. FALSE   C. TRUE   D. FALSE   E. FALSE

The larynx consists of three single cartilages (epiglottis, thyroid and cricoid) and three pairs (cuneiform, corniculate and arytenoid). The external branch of the superior laryngeal nerve supplies the cricothyroid muscle.

QUESTION 28

A. FALSE B. TRUE C. FALSE D. TRUE E. FALSE

Asbestos is linked with the pleural tumour, a mesothelioma. Squamous cell carcinoma is the most common and has the best prognosis. Small cell tumours have the worst prognosis. Some tumours can secrete peptide hormones, e.g. PTH, ACTH and the APUD analogues.

QUESTION 29

A. FALSE B. FALSE C. TRUE D. FALSE E. FALSE

Rheumatic fever is the most common precedent to mitral valve stenosis, and in these cases is more common in women. There is left atrial hypertrophy, and this may develop into pulmonary hypertension and right heart failure. The most common complication is atrial fibrillation with subsequent embolic episodes. Endocarditis is more commonly associated with aortic disease.

QUESTION 30

A. TRUE B. FALSE C. FALSE D. TRUE E. FALSE

Smoking, diabetes, high low density lipoprotein plasma cholesterol and hypertension are the main risk factors for atherosclerosis. Hyperfibrinogenaemia, high plasma factors VIIc and VIIIc are also implicated.

QUESTION 31

A. TRUE B. TRUE C. FALSE D. TRUE E. FALSE

Venous gangrene is a rare condition in which peripheral venous return is acutely occluded despite good arterial supply. It may be due to increased blood viscosity caused by an underlying malignancy or polycythemia. Deeper layers are sometimes spared.

QUESTION 32

A. TRUE B. TRUE C. FALSE D. FALSE E. TRUE

Four layer compression bandaging provides gradually decreasing pressure from the ankle to the knee. It should be avoided in the presence of arterial disease and diabetic arterial disease. Overtight bandaging may result in ischaemia or local pressure necrosis.

QUESTION 33

A. FALSE B. FALSE C. TRUE D. FALSE E. TRUE

Gout is a disorder of purine metabolism. Allopurinol is contraindicated in the acute phase. Deposition of uric acid crystals in the kidney tubules can result in renal failure. Calcium pyrophosphate crystals are seen in pseudogout.

QUESTION 34

A. TRUE B. TRUE C. FALSE D. TRUE E. FALSE

Osteomalacia (rickets in children) is associated with disorders of vitamin D synthesis or function, resulting in inadequate mineralisation of the collagen matrix.

QUESTION 35

A. TRUE   B. FALSE   C. TRUE   D. TRUE   E. TRUE

Fracture complications can be immediate or delayed. Myositis ossificans involves calcification of soft tissues around a fracture causing joint stiffness. Volkmann's contracture results from a forearm compartment syndrome, and Sudek's atrophy is a reflex sympathetic dystrophy following wrist fractures.

QUESTION 36

A. FALSE   B. FALSE   C. FALSE   D. FALSE   E. TRUE

QUESTION 37

A. TRUE   B. FALSE   C. FALSE   D. FALSE   E. FALSE

Most duodenal perforations occur on the anterior duodenal surface. The diagnosis is clinical, but air under the diaphragm is only seen in 70% of cases, and therefore its absence does not exclude perforation. Endoscopy is not indicated to confirm this diagnosis.

QUESTION 38

A. TRUE   B. TRUE   C. TRUE   D. TRUE   E. TRUE

Very high levels of gastrin are consistent with gastrin secreting tumours as occur in Zollinger-Ellison syndrome, which may form part of a MEN I syndrome. Raised gastrin is also seen in a number of other conditions.

QUESTION 39

A. TRUE   B. FALSE   C. TRUE   D. TRUE   E. TRUE

Acute prostatitis can be bacterial, viral or chemical through inadvertent oily phenol injection. If bacterial, spread is usually haematogenous from a distant source. This can then give rise to systemic sepsis.

QUESTION 40

A. TRUE   B. FALSE   C. TRUE   D. TRUE   E. TRUE

Any lesion that can obstruct both ureters can give rise to hydronephrosis. This also includes the bladder neck and urethra.

QUESTION 41

A. TRUE   B. TRUE   C. TRUE   D. FALSE   E. TRUE

Initially after injury, the bladder becomes distended without pain and therefore requires drainage. Long term after injury, the bladder becomes flaccid. Treatment options are permanent indwelling catheter, intermittent self-catheterisation, or urinary diversion. Stones may form as a result of immobility and give rise to infections.

QUESTION 42

A. FALSE   B. FALSE   C. TRUE   D. TRUE   E. TRUE

Papillary carcinoma of the thyroid is common in iodine rich areas and has highest frequency in the under 40 age group. Spread is mainly lymphatic but vascular invasion does occur. Orphan Annie cells have pale cytoplasm with inclusions giving a distinctive appearance.

QUESTION 43

A. FALSE   B. TRUE   C. TRUE   D. FALSE   E. TRUE

Solitary parathyroid adenoma account for 90% of cases of primary hyperparathyroidism. Parathyroid hyperplasia is associated with the MEN syndromes. Osteitis fibrocystica and kidney stones can form part of the presentation. Chvostek's sign is positive in hypocalcaemia.

QUESTION 44

A. FALSE   B. FALSE   C. FALSE   D. TRUE   E. TRUE

Primary hyperaldosteronism is usually due to an adenoma of the adrenal cortex secreting excess mineralocorticoids. This differs from secondary hyperaldosteronism in which renin is raised due inadequate kidney perfusion. There is loss of potassium and hydrogen ions with a rise in serum sodium.

QUESTION 45

A. FALSE   B. TRUE   C. FALSE   D. FALSE   E. FALSE

A bloody discharge suggests malignancy or an intraduct papilloma. Other conditions may give rise to a serous or milky discharge. Mondor's disease is thrombophlebitis of superficial veins over the breast of unknown aetiology.

QUESTION 46

A. FALSE   B. TRUE   C. TRUE   D. TRUE   E. FALSE

Puberty, drugs, liver disease and testicular tumours are the most common causes of gynaecomastia. Approximately 1% of all breast cancers occur in men.

QUESTION 47

A. TRUE   B. FALSE   C. FALSE   D. TRUE   E. TRUE

Tamoxifen works primarily by blocking oestrogen receptors on tumour cells, though beneficial effects are also seen in oestrogen receptor negative tumours. There is a increased risk of endometrial cancer in prolonged usage.

QUESTION 48

A. TRUE   B. TRUE   C. FALSE   D. TRUE   E. TRUE

Wilms' tumour may also be associated with other chromosomal abnormalities, and normally presents below the age of 5 years. The older the presentation, the less favourable the prognosis.

QUESTION   49

A. FALSE   B. FALSE   C. FALSE   D. TRUE   E. FALSE

The rate is 1–2%. Most testes lie at the superficial inguinal ring. There is decreased fertility possibly due to higher temperatures and a much increased risk of malignant change, particularly if the testes is intra-abdominal.

QUESTION   50

A. TRUE   B. TRUE   C. FALSE   D. FALSE   E. FALSE

Inguinal hernia are present in up to 5% of infants, with the rate rising to 10% in preterm infants. As in adults , this condition is more common in males. Surgery does not require reinforcement of the posterior wall, but dissection of the sac can put the testicular blood supply at risk. Although the condition is frequently bilateral, routine exploration of the contralateral side is not normally advocated.

Exam 4

QUESTION 1

Anaemia is commonly present in the following groups of patients

A. Insulin dependent diabetics
B. Chronic renal failure
C. Post chemotherapy
D. Chronic obstructive airways disease (COAD)
E. Smokers

QUESTION 2

Myocardial Infarction (MI)

A. In the perioperative period is associated with a 10% mortality
B. Is a relative contraindication to elective surgery within the first 12 months following an MI
C. Shows acute ST segment elevation on the chest leads of a 12 lead ECG soon after an MI
D. Postoperative MI should be treated immediately with streptokinase infusion
E. Is more common in men than women

QUESTION 3

Factors that would indicate a significant risk of post-operative respiratory problems include

A. A FVC (forced vital capacity) of less than 15ml/kg
B. A high FEV1(forced expiratory volume at 1 second)/FVC ratio
C. A high resting respiratory rate
D. A low haemoglobin
E. A high peak expiratory flow rate (PEFR)

QUESTION 4

"Crash" induction of anaesthesia

A. Is contraindicated in pregnancy
B. Is necessary in all emergency/trauma patients
C. Cricoid pressure is used to occlude the oesophagus during tracheal intubation
D. Intravenous anaesthesia is administered
E. Non-depolarising muscle relaxants are rapidly infused

QUESTION 5

Normal general anaesthetic monitoring of a patient undergoing a hernia repair would include

A. Urine output
B. Arterial blood pressure
C. Oxygen saturation
D. Arterial blood gas
E. Central venous pressure

QUESTION 6

In the American Society of Anesthesiologists (ASA) classification of physical status prior to surgery

A. A patient with mild asymptomatic hypertension would be grade I
B. Renal dialysis patient with no other disease is grade III
C. Any patient requiring immediate emergency surgery is automatically grade V
D. A moribund patient not expected to survive 24 hours post-surgery is grade V
E. Grade IV requires impairment of at least two body systems

QUESTION 7

Suitable patients for admission to intensive care unit would include

A. Deteriorating respiratory function and urine output in a 36 year old man with acute pancreatitis despite maximal resuscitation
B. Ruptured abdominal aortic aneurysm in 85 year old man unfit for surgery
C. Deteriorating conscious level post head injury in a 25 year old lady
D. Post hemicolectomy in a 72 year old man with emphysema and renal impairment
E. Severe chest infection in a 70 year old lady with metastatic breast cancer

QUESTION 8

Common complications of Total Parenteral Nutrition (TPN) include

A. Hyperglycaemia
B. Hyperphosphataemia
C. Hypernatraemia
D. Hypermagnesiumia
E. Hyperosmolar diuresis

QUESTION 9

Causes of renal failure include

A. Decreased systemic vascular resistance
B. Jaundice
C. Anaemia
D. Renal artery stenosis
E. Hypovolaemic shock

QUESTION 10

Ciprofloxacin

A. Is a quinolone type anti-biotic
B. Is effective against Pseudomonas infections
C. Is effective against streptoccocal infections
D. Has good anti-anaerobic activity
E. Is used in urinary tract infections

QUESTION 11

Subphrenic abscess

A. May present with a swinging pyrexia
B. Can occur after laproscopic cholecystectomy
C. Can cause weight loss
D. Do not normally require drainage
E. May be associated with a pleural effusion

QUESTION 12

A Kocher incision

A. Is suitable for an open cholecystectomy
B. Is predominantly muscle splitting in nature
C. May put the ilio-inguinal nerve at risk
D. Is closed using two layer chromic catgut
E. Follows Langer's lines

QUESTION 13

The neodynium yttrium aluminium garnet (NdYAG) laser is commonly employed in the following procedures

A. Transitional cell carcinoma of the bladder
B. Pre-cancerous lesions of the cervix
C. Obstructive oesophageal carcinoma
D. Port wine skin lesions
E. Retinal lesions

QUESTION 14

In the mesh repair of an inguinal hernia

A. Damage to the ilio-inguinal nerve may result in sensory loss at the base of the penis
B. The sac is always dissected to its apex
C. The sac is always opened before reduction
D. The lower edge of the mesh is secured to the lacunar ligament
E. The upper edge of the mesh is secured to the conjoint tendon

QUESTION 15

Fat embolism

A. Follows spinal fracture and cord damage
B. Is characterised by raised plasma triglycerides
C. May present with symptoms of a pulmonary embolism
D. May precipitate a coagulopathy
E. If occuring within the limbs should be removed with a Fogarty catheter embolectomy

QUESTION 16

Cardiac tamponade

A. Occurs only after penetrating injuries to the heart
B. Is characterised by arterial hypertension
C. The central venous pressure is raised
D. Should be treated with aspiration using a needle inserted via the second intercostal space, mid-clavicular line
E. Is characterised by increase ECG voltage across all leads

QUESTION 17

The following tumours are sensitive to radiotherapy

A. Malignant melanoma
B. Squamous cell carcinoma of the anus
C. Adenocarcinoma of the oesophagus
D. Seminoma of the testicle
E. Pancreatic carcinoma

QUESTION 18

The following carcinogens have been implicated in the malignancies below

A. Aflatoxin and hepatocellular carcinoma
B. Schistosomiasis and transitional cell carcinoma of the bladder
C. Alcohol and pancreatic carcinoma
D. Infra-red irradiation and malignant melanoma
E. Nitrosamines and gastric carcinoma

QUESTION 19

Principles of a programme in the screening of malignant disease include

A. Screening tests should be invasive to maximise sensitivity
B. There must be a means of treating the disease if diagnosed early
C. Patients should be prepared to take the consequences of diagnosis and further investigations or treatment
D. Should not include people above 60 years old
E. Long term survival benefits should be demonstrated in a screened population as opposed to a non-screened population

QUESTION   20

Side effects of cyclosporin include

- **A.** Nephrotoxicity
- **B.** Alopecia
- **C.** Obesity
- **D.** Gingival Hypertrophy
- **E.** Tremors

QUESTION   21

The following situations may give rise to a increased bleeding tendency

- **A.** Infusions of Hartmann's solution
- **B.** Aspirin
- **C.** Protein C deficiency
- **D.** Jaundice
- **E.** Uraemia

QUESTION   22

The following statements concerning prophylaxis of thrombo–embolic disease are true

- **A.** An appropriate regimen involves enoxaparin 20 mg bd, given subcutaneously
- **B.** Clinically significant thromboembolism occurs in approximately 1% of patients undergoing major surgery
- **C.** Mechanical measures contribute significantly to reduce the incidence of thromboembolism
- **D.** Dextran 70 is widely used to reduce the incidence of postoperative deep vein thrombosis
- **E.** Age >35 years, obesity and malignancy are all significant risk factors for the development of deep vein thrombosis

QUESTION   23

Indications for a tracheostomy include

- **A.** Patients on long term ventilation
- **B.** Post radical neck dissection
- **C.** Post laryngectomy
- **D.** Comatose patients with heavy secretions
- **E.** Pharyngeal pouch

QUESTION 24

Regarding consent for surgery

A. Refusal to give consent for surgery by a fit and mentally sound adult for a life threatening condition is equivalent to assisted suicide

B. Refusal of consent by mentally ill patients is invalid

C. Action without consent may bring a charge of battery against the clinician

D. Consent is implied when the patient assents to the doctors requests during an examination

E. A close relative can give consent on instead of a patient who is seriously ill but competent and refusing treatment

QUESTION 25

The following criteria must exist before a diagnosis of brain death can be made

A. Fixed, dilated pupils unresponsive to light

B. Absent gag reflex with pharyngeal stimulation

C. Neuromuscular drugs should have been stopped for at least twelve hours

D. No eye movement when 20 mls cold water is perfused into the external auditory meatus

E. No motor response from painful stimuli

QUESTION 26

Regarding the parotid gland

A. It is divided into deep and superficial parts by the mandibular nerve

B. The main duct opens in the mouth opposite the second lower molar tooth

C. Is inflamed in Sjogrens syndrome

D. Approximately 15% of salivary gland tumours occur in the parotid

E. The majority of tumours occuring in the parotid are benign

QUESTION 27

Tumours of the salivary gland

A. 10% of submandibular gland tumours are malignant

B. Fine needle aspiration is contraindicated as an investigation

C. Warthins tumours of the parotid show a high malignant potential

D. May arise from pre-existing Sjogren's syndrome

E. May be secondary lesions from the scalp

QUESTION 28

The diaphragm

A. Receives its nerve supply from the phrenic, vagus and intercostal nerves
B. Can give rise to a hernia through the foramen of Morgagni which occurs between the costal and sternal attachments
C. Failure of closure of the pleuroperitoneal canal can give rise to a hernia through the foramen of Bochdalek
D. May cause incarceration of a gastric volvulus
E. Is derived from migratory myotomes derived from the upper thoracic somites

QUESTION 29

The following risk factors are associated with the development of coronary artery disease

A. Diabetes mellitus
B. Hypercholestrolaemia in particular with high levels of HDL (high density lipoproteins)
C. Male sex
D. Hypertension
E. Deletion polymorphism in the ACE (angiotensin-converting enzyme) gene

QUESTION 30

Carotid artery stenosis

A. Can present with amaurosis fugax
B. Is not amenable to surgery if the plaque is ulcerated
C. Complete unilateral occlusion is an indication for urgent surgery
D. The risk of stroke following surgery is greater than 10%
E. Patients who have already had a major stroke are likely to benefit most from surgery

QUESTION 31

Complications of chronic varicose vein disease include

A. Eczema
B. Lipodermatosclerosis
C. Equinus deformity
D. Malignant transformation
E. Deep vein thrombosis

QUESTION 32

Thrombangitis obliterans (Beurger's disease)

A. is most common in oriental women
B. Affects vessels in the head and neck
C. Is associated with smoking
D. Is associated with HLA A9
E. May cause gangrene resulting in amputation

QUESTION 33

Rheumatoid arthritis

A. Is diagnosed in all patients with a positive test for rheumatoid factor
B. Tends to occur unilaterally in the large joints
C. Is more common in men
D. Is characterised by marginal bony erosions on X-rays
E. Subluxation of joints is a late feature

QUESTION 34

Perthes' disease

A. Is also known as coxa plana or pseudocoxalgia
B. Is common in the early teenage years
C. Is more common in boys
D. Abduction and internal rotation are usually limited
E. Should be treated with internal fixation of the femoral head

QUESTION 35

Bone tumours

A. Primary are more common than secondary
B. Primary tumours are characterised by a Bence-Jones proteins in the urine
C. Giant cell lesions can be benign
D. Paget's disease pre-disposes to osteosarcoma
E. Ewings tumour are derived from chondrocytes

QUESTION 36

Inguinal hernia

A. Occur most commonly in young adult males
B. Are indirect if the sac emerges lateral to the inferior epigastric vessels
C. Are most commonly repaired using an absorbable mesh
D. Occur due to a weakness in the external oblique aponeurosis
E. Appear below and lateral to the pubic tubercle

QUESTION 37

Indications for urgent surgery in 75 year old patient with haematemesis include

A. Six units blood transfusion with continued requirements
B. Major rebleed within 48 hours of first
C. Presence of portal hypertension
D. If active arterial bleeding is seen on endoscopy
E. Widespread gastric erosions seen on endoscopy

QUESTION 38

Haemorrhoids

A. Usually present with pain on defecation
B. Represent dilatation of submucosal venous plexuses below the anorectal ring
C. "Third degree" are prolapsed requiring manual reduction
D. Primary and secondary can be treated with injections of oily phenol
E. Predispose to fistula formation

QUESTION 39

Benign prostatic hypertrophy (BPH)

A. Causes narrowing of the prostatic urethra
B. Can precipitate bladder calculi
C. Can present with haematuria
D. Can be treated pharmacologically with a 5-alpha reductase inhibitor
E. The presence of a raised serum prostatic specific antigen (PSA) level is conclusive of prostatic carcinoma

QUESTION 40

A staghorn renal calculus

A. Consists of calcium oxalate
B. Is associated with Proteus mirabilis infection
C. Frequently present with ureteric colic
D. Can cause deterioration of renal function
E. Should not be removed by extra-corporeal shock wave lithotripsy (ESWL) alone

QUESTION 41

Detrusor muscle overactivity

A. Can result from diabetes
B. May occur in the absence of any neurological abnormality
C. Results in stress incontinence
D. Urodynamic studies indicate high detrusor pressures at low bladder volumes
E. Can be treated medically with anti-cholinergic drugs

QUESTION 42

Anaplastic carcinoma of the thyroid

A. Is very aggressive
B. Occurs in elderly patients
C. Is more common in men
D. Consists histologically of Hurthle cells
E. Arises on the background of Hashimoto's thyroiditis

QUESTION 43

Carcinoid syndrome

A. Can occur in any advanced disseminated malignancy of GI origin
B. Symptoms include diarrhoea
C. The main circulating hormone is vasopressin
D. Diagnosis is confirmed by raised levels of VMA (vanillymandelic acid) in the urine
E. Treatment may include hepatic artery embolisation of secondary deposits

QUESTION 44

Glucocorticoids

A. Are secreted from the zona fasciculata within the adrenal cortex
B. Molecules consist of 21 carbon atoms
C. Cause retention of sodium
D. Inhibit gluconeogenesis
E. Reduce lymphocyte counts

QUESTION 45

The following genetic disorders have been linked to the development of breast cancer

A. Li-Fraumeni syndrome
B. Lynch II syndrome
C. Gardners syndrome
D. Von Hippel-Lindau syndrome
E. Peutz-Jegher syndrome

QUESTION 46

Paget's disease of the nipple

A. Is frequently bilateral
B. Is similar in appearance to eczema
C. Is associated with an underlying intraduct carcinoma
D. Is associated with Phylloides tumour of the breast
E. Is treated with radiotherapy

QUESTION 47

Reconstruction following breast surgery

A. Should not be carried out at the same time as initial surgery
B. Using a latissimus dorsi flap makes use of the thoraco-dorsal neurovascular bundle
C. Using a free transverse rectus abdominus muscle (TRAM) flap requires anastamosis of the inferior epigastric vessels
D. Silicone implants are contraindicated in breast cancer
E. Lymphoedema of the upper limb is a common complication

QUESTION   48

Gastroschisis

  A. Is an abdominal wall defect occuring to the right of the umbilicus
  B. The defect is covered in a peritoneal sac
  C. Is associated with Trisomy 21
  D. Other viscera are frequently involved
  E. The defect size is usually small

QUESTION   49

Hirschsprung's disease

  A. Affects 1 in 5000 births
  B. Is associated with trisomy 21
  C. May be complicated with enterocolitis
  D. Is treated in the first instance with a colostomy or ileostomy
  E. Is associated with increased risk of colo-rectal cancer in the adult

QUESTION   50

Choledochal cysts

  A. Occur in at a rate of approximately 1 in 10 000 births
  B. The commonest type (type I) consists of dilatation of the cystic duct
  C. The presentation triad includes jaundice, pain and an abdominal mass
  D. Simple drainage is normally all that is required
  E. There is a long term risk of increased malignancy

Exam 4: Answers

QUESTION 1

A. FALSE B. TRUE C. TRUE D. FALSE E. FALSE

Chronic diseases and malignancies are associated with anaemia. In respiratory disease the body attempts to compensate through increased red cell production.

QUESTION 2

A. FALSE B. FALSE C. TRUE D. FALSE E. TRUE

Post operative MI is associated with a greater than 40% mortality. Fibrinolytic therapy is contraindicated post-operatively. Risk of a repeat MI associated with surgery is less than 6% (cf no previous MI risk is 0-5%) after six months.

QUESTION 3

A. TRUE B. FALSE C. TRUE D. FALSE E. FALSE

High risk patients for respiratory complications include smokers, asthmatics, COAD patients, obese and elderly. Pre-operative optimisation of lung function is essential, smoking should be stopped. Post-operative pain control, physiotherapy and early mobilisation are important factors in reducing risk.

QUESTION 4

A. FALSE B. TRUE C. TRUE D. TRUE E. FALSE

Crash induction is used in any situation where there is a risk of aspiration of gastric contents, This includes pregnancy, trauma and emergency non fasted patients. Intravenous anaesthesia (thiopentone) and short acting depolarising muscle relaxant (suxamethonium) are normally used in conjunction with maintained cricoid pressure.

QUESTION 5

A. FALSE B. TRUE C. TRUE D. FALSE E. FALSE

Minor / intermediate surgery of less than one hour requires only basic cardiac and respiratory monitoring unless pre-existing medical pathology is present.

QUESTION 6

A. FALSE   B. TRUE   C. FALSE   D. TRUE   E. FALSE

The ASA classifies a healthy patient as Grade I. Any emergency procedure is given an "E" in addition. Mild systemic disease without functional limitation qualifies as grade II. Severe systemic disease with definite function limitation is grade III. Grade IV represents severe systemic disease which is a constant threat to life.

QUESTION 7

A. TRUE   B. FALSE   C. TRUE   D. TRUE   E. FALSE

Patients admitted to an ITU require organ support and / or close monitoring. There must be a overall chance of favourable outcome to justify this therapy.

QUESTION 8

A. TRUE   B. FALSE   C. TRUE   D. FALSE   E. TRUE

QUESTION 9

A. TRUE   B. TRUE   C. FALSE   D. TRUE   E. TRUE

Renal failure can be precipitated by diminished renal perfusion, glomerular or tubular damage. Hepatorenal failure occurs in jaundiced patients. Decreased renal can occur as a result of decreased circulatory volume (hypovolaemia) or decreased systemic vascular resistance as in septic shock.

QUESTION 10

A. TRUE   B. TRUE   C. FALSE   D. FALSE   E. TRUE

The quinolones represent a new generation of antibiotics.

QUESTION 11

A. TRUE   B. TRUE   C. TRUE   D. FALSE   E. TRUE

Treatment is by image controlled aspiration in the first instance.

QUESTION 12

A. TRUE   B. FALSE   C. FALSE   D. FALSE   E. FALSE

Kocher's incisions are rarely used now. They are associated with weakness of the anterior abdominal wall due to damage of the neurovascular bundles from the lower ribs. Catgut is not used in abdominal wall closure.

QUESTION 13

A. TRUE   B. FALSE   C. TRUE   D. FALSE   E. TRUE

CO_2 lasers are used to treat early cervical lesions. Ruby laser light is effective in the treatment of superficial skin lesions.

QUESTION   14

A. TRUE   B. FALSE   C. FALSE   D. FALSE   E. TRUE

Inguinal hernia may be direct or indirect. Direct hernial sacs do not usually require opening unless there is concern about the contents. An indirect sac that enters the scrotum is not usually dissected beyond the mid-inguinal point in case of testicular ischaemia.

QUESTION   15

A. FALSE   B. TRUE   C. TRUE   D. TRUE   E. FALSE

Fat embolism can follow fractures of long bones, releasing bone marrow, which in addition to increased fat and lipid, mobilisation, increased synthesis and reduced uptake as part of the trauma response raises the level of circulating lipids. This can have several severe systemic effects, including ARDS, DIC, and eventually multi-organ failure.

QUESTION   16

A. FALSE   B. FALSE   C. TRUE   D. FALSE   E. FALSE

Cardiac tamponade can occur after both penetrating and blunt injuries to the chest, and is charac-terised by, hypotension, Kussmaul sign, raised JVP, muffled heart sounds and decreased voltages in all ECG leads.

QUESTION   17

A. FALSE   B. TRUE   C. FALSE   D. TRUE   E. FALSE

Squamous cell carcinoma respond well to radiotherapy. Adenocarcinoma show a variable but generally poor response.

QUESTION   18

A. TRUE   B. FALSE   C. FALSE   D. FALSE   E. TRUE

Schistosomiasis is linked with squamous cell carcinoma of the bladder. Alcohol is linked with oesophageal and gastric cancers, and ultraviolet light exposure increases risk of malignant melanoma.

QUESTION   19

A. FALSE   B. TRUE   C. TRUE   D. FALSE   E. TRUE

A screening programme aims to improve survival from a disease if diagnosed early, i.e before it becomes symptomatic. Therefore, there has to be a method of treatment available for the early disease, even if there are no symptoms. Patients must be compliant to screening, which means low risk tests that have high sensitivity and specificity. At present the UK breast screening programme is under con-tinued evaluation. Screening has been suggested for prostatic, ovarian and colorectal carcinoma, but have not been approved.

QUESTION   20

A. TRUE   B. FALSE   C. FALSE   D. TRUE   E. TRUE

Other complications include skin problems, hypertension, haemolytic anaemia and malignant change.

QUESTION 21

A. FALSE   B. TRUE   C. FALSE   D. TRUE   E. TRUE

Hartmann's solution is unlikely to interfere with clotting, unlike infusions of tissue expanders containing dextran. Aspirin and uraemia can affect platelet function, and jaundice reduces hepatic absorption of vitamin K. Protein C deficiency causes increased clotting tendency.

QUESTION 22

A. FALSE   B. TRUE   C. TRUE   D. FALSE   E. FALSE

QUESTION 23

A. TRUE   B. FALSE   C. TRUE   D. TRUE   E. FALSE

Tracheostomy reduces anatomical dead space and makes ventilation and clearance of secretions easier.

QUESTION 24

A. FALSE   B. FALSE   C. TRUE   D. TRUE   E. FALSE

No adult can give consent on behalf of another, if the patient concerned is mentally competent, even if the illness is life threatening. Refusal to give consent does not amount to suicide if the patient did not bring about the cause of disease themselves. A patient who has a mental disorder can refuse consent if the patient is mentally "capable" of doing so. Implied consent is taken when a patient complies with the clinician's requests, having been fully informed in advance, although this may be difficult to prove later without written evidence.

QUESTION 25

A. TRUE   B. FALSE   C. FALSE   D. TRUE   E. TRUE

An absent gag reflex must be assessed with bronchial stimulation via a tracheal catheter. Neuromuscular drugs should have been stopped for 24 hours at least before assessment can be made.

QUESTION 26

A. FALSE   B. FALSE   C. TRUE   D. FALSE   E. TRUE

The parotid gland is divided by the facial nerve and its branches. The duct opens opposite the upper second molar. The majority of salivary gland tumours occur in the parotid, the majority of these are benign, and the majority of the are pleomorphic adenoma.

QUESTION 27

A. FALSE   B. FALSE   C. FALSE   D. TRUE   E. TRUE

50% of submandibular tumours and 10% of submandibular tumours are malignant. Malignant lesions include adenocarcinoma, acinic cell carcinoma, adenoid cystic carcinoma, squamous cell carcinoma, and lymphoma (which may occur on the background of Sjögren's syndrome). The salivary glands may be sites for secondary spread from the scalp and oral cavity.

QUESTION 28

A. FALSE   B. TRUE   C. TRUE   D. TRUE   E. FALSE

The diaphragm is embryologically derived from the cervical myotomes, and brings its nerve supply with it. The foramen of Morgagni lies anteriorly and that of Bochdalek posteriorly. A gastric volvulus can become incarcerated and ischaemic, particularly in the presence of an pre-existing hiatus hernia.

QUESTION 29

A. TRUE   B. FALSE   C. TRUE   D. TRUE   E. TRUE

Hyperlipidaemia in the presence of low levels of HDL is a strong risk factor. Possession of an ACE gene polymorphic marker (D) is a risk factor, and those with a DD genotype are at higher risk.

QUESTION 30

A. TRUE   B. FALSE   C. FALSE   D. FALSE   E. FALSE

Surgery in carotid artery stenosis has been shown to be beneficial in symptomatic patients with occlusion of 70-99%. Complete occlusion (perfusion of brain via circle of Willis) and established hemispheric damage are contraindications for further intervention. Ulcerated plaques tend to give more symptoms due to greater embolic formation.

QUESTION 31

A. TRUE   B. TRUE   C. TRUE   D. TRUE   E. FALSE

Equinus deformity occurs following prolonged walking on toes to relieve pain. This can then result in permanent Achilles tendon shortening. Squamous cell carcinoma can occur in the base of chronic venous ulcers (Marjolin's ulcer).

QUESTION 32

A. FALSE   B. FALSE   C. TRUE   D. TRUE   E. TRUE

Beurgers's disease is a progressive arterial obliteration of medium sized vessels of unknown aetiology. It affects men who are invariably smokers and is more common in eastern countries. treatment is initially through stopping smoking and possibly anticoagulation.

QUESTION 33

A. FALSE   B. FALSE   C. FALSE   D. TRUE   E. TRUE

Rheumatoid arthritis is a symmetrical polyarthritis most commonly affecting the proximal joints of the hands and feet. It is autoimmune inflammatory in nature, although rheumatoid factor is only present in 80% of cases, and is not diagnostic alone. It occurs three times more commonly in women

QUESTION 34

A. TRUE   B. FALSE   C. TRUE   D. TRUE   E. FALSE

Perthes disease is avascular necrosis of the femoral head of unknown aetiology. The age group affected is 4-8 years. Treatment is with bed rest and traction in the first instance.

QUESTION 35

A. FALSE   B. FALSE   C. TRUE   D. TRUE   E. FALSE

Primary bone tumours are rare. Bence-Jones proteins are seen in multiple myeloma. Giant cell tumours, one third are benign, one third locally invasive, one third metastasize. Ewing's tumour arise from vascular endothelium.

QUESTION 36

A. FALSE   B. TRUE   C. FALSE   D. FALSE   E. FALSE

QUESTION 37

A. TRUE   B. TRUE   C. FALSE   D. TRUE   E. FALSE

Patients who have a high probability of responding to medical management should be considered for surgery. In elderly patients the threshold for surgery is much lower, and large transfusion requirements, re-bleed, or an aggressive lesion on endoscopy are indications for surgery. Presence of portal hypertension, oesphageal varices or lesions not amenable to surgery are contraindications to immediate intervention.

QUESTION 38

A. FALSE   B. FALSE   C. TRUE   D. TRUE   E. FALSE

Haemorrhoids are common lesions resulting from dilatation of submucosal venous plexuses from above the anorectal ring. The most common symptom is painless bleeding. Discomfort can occur if they are prolapsed or another lesion is present.

QUESTION 39

A. TRUE   B. TRUE   C. TRUE   D. TRUE   E. FALSE

Benign enlargement of the prostate causes distortion of the urethra and bladder neck. Stasis of urine and engorgement of the prostatic venous plexus may give symptoms of bladder calculi and haematuria. Beta-blockers and 5 alpha reductase inhibitors are the mainstay of pharmacological treatment. Raised PSA is not an absolute indicator of carcinoma.

QUESTION 40

A. FALSE   B. TRUE   C. FALSE   D. TRUE   E. TRUE

Staghorn calculi are composed of calcium, phosphate and magnesium ammonia phosphate. Production is enhaced by Proteus infection which alkalinises the urine. Symptoms of renal colic are rare, due to it size. Common complains are of recurrent infections or the presence of a mass. Large stones will inhibit renal function, and are difficult to remove by ESWL.

QUESTION 41

A. FALSE B. TRUE C. FALSE D. TRUE E. TRUE

Detrusor overactivity may be primary, or secondary to a neurological or intravesical lesion. Symptomatically patients have frequency and urge incontinence.

QUESTION 42

A. TRUE B. TRUE C. FALSE D. FALSE E. FALSE

This is a rapidly invasive tumour occurring in elderly patients with high mortality. It consists of poorly differentiated cells. Hashimoto thyroiditis may precede lymphoma of the thyroid.

QUESTION 43

A. FALSE B. TRUE C. FALSE D. FALSE E. TRUE

Carcinoid syndrome consist of flushing, diarrhoea, bronchoconstriction and right heart valve disease. This due to the secretion of serotonin and other hormones from the tumours. Carcinoid syndrome rarely occurs in the absence of hepatic metastases if the primary lesion is in the gut as the liver can metabolise these hormone. Raised levels of 5-hydroxyindoleacetic acid are found in the urine. Destruction of hepatic metastases by enucleation or embolisation is a treatment strategy.

QUESTION 44

A. TRUE B. TRUE C. TRUE D. FALSE E. TRUE

The glucocorticoids consist of cortisol and corticosterone. The main effects are in protein, glucose and fat metabolism. There is a slight mineralocorticoid effect, and also an anti-inflammatory effect.

QUESTION 45

A. TRUE B. TRUE C. FALSE D. FALSE E. FALSE

Li-Fraumeni syndrome is due to loss or mutation of the p53 gene. Lynch II syndrome is autosomal dominant condition linked to breast and ovarian cancers.

QUESTION 46

A. FALSE B. TRUE C. TRUE D. FALSE E. FALSE

Paget's disease is determined histologically by specific cells within the nipple. These may have arisen from an underlying carcinoma and migrated along the ducts, or formed within the skin of the nipple. If a lump is present, then these patients are most likely to have invasive cancer. Formal surgical excision with a mastectomy and axillary clearance is normally carried out.

QUESTION 47

A. FALSE B. TRUE C. TRUE D. FALSE E. FALSE

Immediate breast reconstruction is becoming a more popular choice amongst women with breast cancer. It can also be carried out at a later date using a variety of techniques, including tissue expanders, implants and flaps. Lymphoedema is not a specific complication of reconstruction.

QUESTION   48

A. TRUE   B. FALSE   C. FALSE   D. FALSE   E. TRUE

Gastroschisis defect is not covered in a peritoneal sac and therefore exposes the bowel to amniotic fluid damage. There is atresia of the bowel but other viscera are not normally involved. It is not associated with any syndromes.

QUESTION   49

A. TRUE   B. TRUE   C. TRUE   D. TRUE   E. FALSE

There is a slightly higher incidence in males, and a familial tendency.

QUESTION   50

A. FALSE   B. FALSE   C. FALSE   D. FALSE   E. FALSE

This is a very rare condition (1 in 100 000 births)and can present late in adults. It is classified into five types, type I, a dilation of the common bile duct being the most common. Simple drainage is not usually adequate, and formal biliary reconstruction is required.

Exam 5

QUESTION 1

A twelve lead electrocardiogram (ECG)

A. Is routinely performed in all adults undergoing general anaesthetic
B. Shows a prolonged QT interval in the presence of hypercalcaemia
C. Commonly shows a right axis deviation in pulmonary embolism
D. The QRS complex is exaggerated in cardiac tamponade
E. Shows large Q waves following a myocardial infarction

QUESTION 2

Insulin dependant diabetic patients

A. May suffer "silent" myocardial infarction post surgery.
B. Have a higher risk of wound infection
C. Have a higher incidence of deep vein thrombosis
D. Have a higher incidence of kidney disease
E. May have deranged clotting function

QUESTION 3

The American Society of Anaesthesiologists (ASA) classification of fitness of patients for surgery includes the following

A. ASA 1 where there is no organic, physiological, biochemical or psychiatric disturbance
B. ASA 3 where there is mild to moderate systemic disturbance which does not limit normal activity
C. ASA 4 where there are severe life-threatening systemic disorders
D. ASA 5 where the patient is moribund with little chance of recovery
E. ASA E where the letter E after a particular classification denotes an emergency operation

QUESTION 4

Side effects of halothane include

A. Tachycardia
B. Raised intracranial pressure
C. Renal failure
D. Peripheral vasoconstriction
E. Hepatic dysfunction

QUESTION 5

Spinal anaesthesia

A. Perforates the dura and arachnoid mater
B. Acts rapidly
C. Requires high maintenance infusion doses
D. Is contra-indicated in patients with poor respiratory function
E. May result in a CSF leak

QUESTION 6

Local anaesthesia

A. Only affects sensory nerve fibres
B. Is very effective for incision and drainage of cutaneous abscesses
C. Must be injected into the tissues to become effective
D. In high doses can cause convulsions and bradycardia
E. Acts by blocking the fast sodium channel in neuronal membranes

QUESTION 7

Pulmonary capillary wedge pressure (PCWP)

A. Is measured using a CVP line
B. Corresponds to left atrial pressure
C. Is raised in pulmonary oedema
D. Is used to estimate the systemic venous resistance
E. Is used to assess arterial oxygenation

QUESTION 8

Enteral feeding

A. Can be administered by a fine bore naso-gastric tube
B. Is contraindicated in patients with neurological disease
C. Should only be used if TPN is not possible
D. Is contraindicated in ventilated patients
E. Bolus infusions are preferred to mimic meals

QUESTION 9

Postoperative fluid management of the surgical patient should

A. Include administration of 40 - 60 mmol of potassium in the first 24 hours
B. Account for insensible losses of up to 1500 ml if the patient is septic
C. Include packed red blood cells if the haematocrit falls below 40%
D. Aim to provide at least 1000 calories for the first three postoperative days
E. Be increased if the central venous pressure falls below 8 cm H_2O

QUESTION   10

Pseudomembranous colitis

A. Is caused by overgrowth of Clostridium perfringens in the large bowel
B. Can be caused by cephalosporin use
C. Can result in toxic megacolon if untreated
D. Is treated by intravenous vancomycin
E. Commonly presents with rectal bleeding

QUESTION   11

Hepatitis infection

A. Type C often rapidly progresses to fulminant hepatic failure
B. Non A non B type rarely progresses to fulminant hepatic failure
C. Type B is highly infective following needlestick injuries
D. Type D cannot exist alone
E. Type A may predispose to hepatocellular carcinoma

QUESTION   12

Risks associated with laparoscopic surgery include

A. Visceral perforation
B. Conducted diathermy injury
C. Port-site hernia
D. Hypercapnia
E. Pneumothorax

QUESTION   13

Surgical dressings

A. Should have anti-bacterial properties
B. Prevent gaseous exchange
C. Should absorb discharging fluids
D. Should be difficult to remove
E. Should be odourless

QUESTION   14

An ileostomy

A. Typically produces 1500 - 2000 ml small intestinal content per day
B. May be associated with vitamin B_{12} deficiency
C. Is often fashioned following panproctocolectomy perfomed for inflammatory bowel disease
D. Should preferably be designed as a spout as this promotes the bowel contents to become more formed in nature
E. Is associated with an increased incidence of gallstones and renal calculi

QUESTION 15

Spinal cord injury

- A. May cause widespread vasoconstriction
- B. Paralysis respiration if the level of damage is at the cervico-thoracic junction
- C. Is often associated with other systemic injuries
- D. Presents with a sensory cut off and rigid paralysis below the level of injury
- E. May cause hypothermia

QUESTION 16

Burn injuries

- A. If full thickness are normally sensitive to pin prick
- B. Affecting a whole lower limb in a child will represent approximately 18% surface area
- C. Are associated with Pseudomonas infections
- D. Is associated with a high mortality in the elderly
- E. Are associated with nitrous oxide toxicity

QUESTION 17

The following malignancies commonly metastasise to bone

- A. Papillary carcinoma of the thyroid
- B. Carcinoma of the breast
- C. Carcinoma of the prostate
- D. Malignant melanoma
- E. Squamous cell carcinoma of the penis

QUESTION 18

The following are common side effects of chemotherapy

- A. Nausea and vomiting
- B. Alopecia
- C. Mucositis
- D. Intestinal strictures
- E. Infertility

QUESTION 19

The following statements apply to the treatment of cancer

- A. Brachytherapy involves the use of liquid nitrogen in the local treatment of malignant disease
- B. Hyperbaric oxygen has been used as a radiosensitizer in radiation therapy
- C. Photodynamic therapy can be used in the treatment of brain tumours
- D. Neoadjuvant therapy is the application of new therapeutic strategies in the management of cancer
- E. Systemic chemotherapeutic agents may fail to cross the blood-brain barrier

QUESTION   20

Graft rejection following renal transplant

- A. If hyperacute is T-cell mediated
- B. If hyperacute is treated with high dose steroids
- C. May present with tenderness over the graft
- D. Is reduced if the doner kidney is irradiated
- E. Chronic rejection occurs over many months and involves T-cells and humoral antibodies

QUESTION   21

Haemoglobin

- A. Consists of two chains of polypeptides with a central haem molecule
- B. The iron is in the ferric (Fe^{3+}) form and surrounded by tetrapyrrole ring
- C. Free in serum is bound to haptoglobin
- D. Free in serum can precipitate renal failure
- E. Affinity to oxygen is increase with rising pH

QUESTION   22

The following are characteristic features of malignant tumours

- A. Pleomorphism
- B. Anaplasia
- C. Metaplasia
- D. Reactive hyperplasia in local lymph nodes
- E. Ulceration

QUESTION   23

Overdose of the following drugs give rise to the typical symptoms and signs

- A. Iron and gastric haemorrhage
- B. Salicylates and tinnitus
- C. Opiates and dilated pupils
- D. Carbon monoxide and perioral parasthesia
- E. Phenothiazines and dyskinesia

QUESTION   24

Principles of the Hippocratic Oath include

- A. To do no harm
- B. To assist the termination of seriously ill patients
- C. To maintain the patients confidentiality
- D. Not to abuse professional relationships
- E. To assist in abortion if requested

QUESTION   25

The following statements about the Glasgow Coma Scale (GCS) are accurate

A. GCS 15-13 is regarded as a minor head injury
B. GCS of 12 or less is an indication for an urgent CT scan
C. GCS of 1-3 is regarded as a very serious head injury
D. Localisation to pain scores three points
E. Eye opening to speech scores three points

QUESTION   26

Branchial cysts

A. Are also known as "cystic hygroma"
B. Are embryological remnants of the first branchial cleft
C. Are lined with squamous epithelium
D. Aspirate contains cholesterol crystals
E. Are located just to the posterior border of sternomastoid

QUESTION   27

The following are well recognised complications after surgery to the head and neck

A. Gustatory sweating after superficial parotidectomy
B. Sialorrhoea (dribbling from the angle of the mouth) after excision of the submandibular gland
C. Exposure keratitis after parotid surgery
D. Horners syndrome after total parotidectomy
E. Shoulder drop and weakness of the deltopectoral girdle after radical lymph node dissection of the neck

QUESTION   28

The following lesions occur in the anterior mediastinum

A. Dermoid cyst
B. Retrosternal goitre
C. Teratomatous thymic tumour
D. Neurofibroma
E. Sarcoid related lymphadenopathy

QUESTION   29

Severe cases of the following conditions may potentially be suitable for heart-lung transplantation

A. Fibrosing alveolitis
B. Pneumocystis carnii pneumonia
C. Sarcoidosis
D. Cystic fibrosis
E. Small cell lung cancer

QUESTION 30

Thrombolytic therapy

A. Is of little benefit in graft thrombosis
B. Is contraindicated in popliteal aneurysm thrombosis
C. Tissue plasminogen activator (TPA) is most commonly used for peripheral thrombosis
D. Should be given as a bolus dose for peripheral thrombosis
E. Complications include distal embolisation

QUESTION 31

Secondary unilateral lymphoedema may be caused by

A. Chronic tuberculosis
B. Filariasis
C. Milroy's disease
D. Nephrotic syndrome
E. Advanced malignancy

QUESTION 32

Factors which lead to an increase in blood viscosity include

A. Polycythaemia
B. Hypofibrinogenaemia
C. Leukaemia
D. Cryoglobinaemia
E. Dehydration

QUESTION 33

Osteonecrosis of the femoral head is associated with

A. Christmas disease
B. Gauchers disease
C. Sickle cell disease
D. Caisson disease
E. Renal transplant

QUESTION 34

The following nerve injuries are associated with the symptoms below

A. Low ulnar nerve injury and thenar wasting
B. Lateral popliteal nerve injury and foot drop
C. Median nerve injury and weakness of thumb adduction
D. Upper brachial plexus injury and weakness of shoulder abduction
E. Lower brachial plexus injury and claw hand

QUESTION 35

Congenital dislocation of the hip

A. Affects boys more commonly than girls
B. Is associated with acetabular dysplasia
C. Treatment with splinting hold the hips flexed and abducted
D. There is delayed development of the upper femoral epiphysis
E. Avascular necrosis of the femoral head develops if untreated

QUESTION 36

Achalasia of the oesophagus

A. Is commonly complicated by carcinoma
B. Clinical presentation is of dysphagia being worse to liquids
C. Is due to hyperactivitity of the neural plexus in the distal oesophagus
D. Is characterised by a "birds beak" oesophagus
E. Is associated with Systemic Lupus Erythromatosis

QUESTION 37

Sequalae of portal hypertension may include

A. Oesophageal and gastric varices
B. Ascites
C. Caput medusae
D. Pancreatitis
E. Haemorrhoids

QUESTION 38

Conditions which may result in a short gut syndrome in adults include

A. Ulcerative colitis
B. Crohns disease
C. Necrotizing enterocolitis
D. Superior mesenteric artery occlusion
E. Tuberculosis

QUESTION 39

Urethral strictures

A. When caused by gonococcal infection occurs at the penoscrotal junction
B. When are multiple, the deepest is usually the narrowest
C. May result in the formation of a urethral divericulum
D. Tend to occur in elderly patients
E. May occur following childbirth in females

QUESTION 40

Adenocarcinoma of the kidney

A. Is also known as a clear cell tumour
B. Arises in the medulla of the kidney
C. Is more common in men
D. Is associated with polycythaemia
E. Commonly metastasises to liver

QUESTION 41

Adenocarcinoma of the kidney

A. Most commonly occurs in women
B. Responds well to chemotherapy
C. May present with a pathological fracture
D. Arises in the glomeruli
E. May be associated with a right sided varicocele

QUESTION 42

Medullary carcinoma of the thyroid

A. Is familial in over 80% of cases
B. Secrete Carcinoembryonic antigen (CEA)
C. Occur in the MEN type I syndrome
D. Frequently metastasis via blood to bone
E. Frequently invades locally

QUESTION 43

Carcinoid tumours

A. Only occur in the gastro-intestinal tract
B. Secrete large amounts of 5-hydroxyindoleacetic acid (5-HIAA)
C. The most common site of tumour is the appendix and distal small bowel
D. The five year survival rate with hepatic metastases is less than 5%
E. May occur as part of a multiple endocrine neoplasia syndrome (MEN)

QUESTION 44

Concerning acute pancreatitis

A. No aetiological factor may be identified in up to 20% of patients
B. May be associated with a normal amylase concentration
C. May be secondary to pancreatic carcinoma
D. Evidence of pancreatic necrosis on CT scan is an indication for necrosectomy
E. If gallstones are implicated as an aetiological factor, laparoscopic cholecystectomy should be performed 3-6 months after complete resolution of the inflammatory process

QUESTION 45

Poor prognosis in breast cancer is associated with

A. Vascular invasion
B. Oestrogen receptor positive
C. Progesterone receptor positive
D. Low grade tumour
E. Lobular type breast cancer

QUESTION 46

Phylloides tumour of the breast

A. Is a transformation of smooth muscle cells within the ducts
B. Consist histologically of epithelial and stromal components
C. Is invasive in the majority of cases
D. Are sensitive to chemotherapy
E. Lymph node spread is rare

QUESTION 47

Nipple discharge

A. Which is blood-stained is always due to breast cancer
B. May be physiological
C. May be bilateral in patients with prolactinaemia
D. Is common in patients with Mondor's disease
E. Due to an intraductal papilloma may require a microdochectomy

QUESTION 48

Biliary atresia

A. Presents with persistant unconjugated hyperbilirubinaemia
B. Affects approximately 1 in 10 000 births
C. Is associated with other GI tract anomalies
D. Type I affects the common hepatic duct
E. Will progress to cirrhosis and liver failure

QUESTION 49

Neuroblastoma

A. Are derived from neural crest cells which would form part of the parasympathetic nervous system normally
B. May present with a Horner's syndrome
C. Increased levels of urinary vanillylmandelic acid are found
D. Frequently invades the inferior vena cava
E. Tumours may extend to within the spinal canal

QUESTION 50

The following statements are true

A. Pyloric atresia is treated by resection and anastomosis
B. Duodenal atresia is commonly associated with Downs syndrome
C. Meconium ileus occurs in approximately 50% of children with cystic fibrosis
D. Neonatal intestinal obstruction is characterised by bilious vomiting, abdominal distension and failure to pass meconium
E. Anorectal atresia is more common in boys than girls

Exam 5: Answers

QUESTION 1

A. FALSE   B. FALSE   C. TRUE   D. FALSE   E. TRUE

ECG are normally indicated in adults over 40, or those with a history of cardiac problems. Hypocalcaemia and hypokalaemia prolong the QT interval. Right axis deviation, right bundle branch block, and a "SI, QIII, TIII" pattern is commonly associated pulmonary embolism. Cardiac tamponade decreases all voltages, and large Q waves follow myocardial infarction.

QUESTION 2

A. TRUE   B. TRUE   C. FALSE   D. TRUE   E. FALSE

Cardiac and renal problems develop with longstanding diabetes. There is also a greater susceptibility to local infections.

QUESTION 3

A. TRUE   B. FALSE   C. TRUE   D. TRUE   E. TRUE

QUESTION 4

A. FALSE   B. TRUE   C. FALSE   D. FALSE   E. TRUE

Halothane is an inhalational anaesthetic. As with other agents this causes cardiorespiratory depression, peripheral and cerebral vasodilation. There is a relative reduction in hepatic blood flow, and the drug is metabolised in the liver which can cause altered function. In rare cases, hepatic necrosis may occur.

QUESTION 5

A. TRUE   B. TRUE   C. FALSE   D. FALSE   E. TRUE

Spinal anaesthesia is a form of local block, in which opioids and / or local anaesthetic is injected into the subarachnoid space. It is most useful inpatients unable to tolerate a general anaesthetic due to poor respiratory or cardiac function.

QUESTION 6

A. FALSE   B. FALSE   C. FALSE   D. TRUE   E. TRUE

QUESTION 7

A. FALSE   B. TRUE   C. TRUE   D. TRUE   E. FALSE

PCWP is normally measured using a Swann-Ganz catheter, which gives a more accurate idea of left atrial pressure than a simple CVP line. Using the Fick principle, cardiac output and hence systemic venous resistance are calculated.

QUESTION 8

A. TRUE   B. FALSE   C. FALSE   D. FALSE   E. FALSE

Enteral nutrition is contraindicated only when the GI tract is completely non-functional or non accessible. Ventilated / neurological patients have a higher risk of aspiration, and so PEG or naso-jejunal feeding is preferred. Continuous overnight infusion is associated with less side-effects and problems.

QUESTION 9

A. FALSE   B. TRUE   C. FALSE   D. FALSE   E. FALSE

QUESTION 10

A. FALSE   B. TRUE   C. FALSE   D. FALSE   E. FALSE

Pseudomembranous colitis is due to overgrowth of *Clostridium difficile* often as a result of antibiotic overuse. It presents with diarrhoea, and is treated with oral metronidazole or oral vancomycin.

QUESTION 11

A. FALSE   B. FALSE   C. TRUE   D. TRUE   E. FALSE

Healthcare workers should be vaccinated for hepatitis B.

QUESTION 12

A. TRUE   B. TRUE   C. TRUE   D. FALSE   E. TRUE

Risks of laparoscopic surgery occur from creating a pneumoperitoneum, from incorrect identification of anatomical structures and excessive use of diathermy causing conduction or capacitance injuries.

QUESTION 13

A. FALSE   B. FALSE   C. TRUE   D. TRUE   E. FALSE

QUESTION 14

A. FALSE   B. TRUE   C. TRUE   D. FALSE   E. TRUE

QUESTION 15

A. FALSE B. FALSE C. TRUE D. FALSE E. TRUE

Spinal shock produces widespread peripheral vasodilation, resulting in hypovolaemia and hypothermia, which may exacerbate other injuries. Respiratory function is switched off if the level of injury is at C3/C4 which affects the phrenic nerve cells. Flaccid paralysis off muscles occurs below the level of injury.

QUESTION 16

A. FALSE B. FALSE C. TRUE D. TRUE E. FALSE

Full thickness injuries have no sensation. Lower limb represent less than 18% of surface area in children, compensated with increased upper limb and head areas as compared to adults. Carbon monoxide toxicity and infection with *Staph. aureus* and *Pseudomonas* are associated with burn injuries. Mortality is highest in the under 2 years and over 70 age groups.

QUESTION 17

A. FALSE B. TRUE C. TRUE D. FALSE E. FALSE

Follicular carcinoma of the thyroid in addition to breast, prostate, kidney and lung primaries are the most frequent tumours going to bone.

QUESTION 18

A. TRUE B. TRUE C. TRUE D. FALSE E. TRUE

Other side-effects include bone marrow suppression and increased long term risk of leukaemia.

QUESTION 19

A. FALSE B. TRUE C. TRUE D. FALSE E. TRUE

QUESTION 20

A. FALSE B. TRUE C. TRUE D. FALSE E. TRUE

Hyperacute rejection occurs if preformed antibodies are present. Acute rejection occurs over a course of days and is T-cell activated. Treatment is increased immunosuppression in the first instance, but if this fails then the graft may have to be removed.

QUESTION 21

A. FALSE B. FALSE C. TRUE D. TRUE E. TRUE

Haemoglobin consists of a central haem molecule with iron in the ferrous (Fe^{2+}) form surrounded by two sets of identical polypeptide chains (i.e. total of four). Excess free haemoglobin can cause endothelial damage and renal failure. Oxygen affinity is decreased with rising hydrogen ion concentration.

QUESTION 22

A. TRUE   B. TRUE   C. FALSE   D. FALSE   E. FALSE

QUESTION 23

A. TRUE   B. TRUE   C. FALSE   D. FALSE   E. TRUE

Opiate overdose produces pinpoint pupils. Carbon monoxide poisoning accounts for a third of UK cases of poisoning and gives rise to headaches, nausea and vomiting, drowsiness, hallucinations and collapse.

QUESTION 24

A. TRUE   B. FALSE   C. TRUE   D. TRUE   E. FALSE

The original Hippocratic Oath has been revised with regards to abortion to "I will maintain the utmost respect for human life from the time of conception."

QUESTION 25

A. TRUE   B. FALSE   C. FALSE   D. FALSE   E. TRUE

The GCS has a minimum of score of 3. A GCS of 12 alone is not an indication for a CT scan.

QUESTION 26

A. FALSE   B. FALSE   C. TRUE   D. TRUE   E. FALSE

Branchial cysts are remnants of the embryololgical second cleft, and normally present as fluctuant swellings anterior to the upper third of the sternomastoid.

QUESTION 27

A. TRUE   B. TRUE   C. TRUE   D. FALSE   E. TRUE

QUESTION 28

A. TRUE   B. TRUE   C. TRUE   D. FALSE   E. FALSE

Lesions of the thyroid and thymus are present in the anterior mediastinum, as are dermoid cysts and teratoma. Neurogenic tumours occur in the posterior mediastinum, and enlarged lymph nodes are central mediastinal structures.

QUESTION 29

A. TRUE   B. FALSE   C. TRUE   D. TRUE   E. FALSE

Normal transplantation rules apply. Therefore presence of malignancy or underlying infection is a contraindication.

QUESTION 30

A. FALSE   B. FALSE   C. TRUE   D. FALSE   E. TRUE

Thrombolytic therapy is useful in acute graft or aneurysm thrombosis. For peripheral disease, continuous or pulse infusions of TPA are administered.

QUESTION 31

A. TRUE   B. TRUE   C. FALSE   D. FALSE   E. TRUE

Milroy's disease is a cause of congenital lymphoedema. Conditions causing hypoproteinaemia or fluid retention result in bilateral oedema.

QUESTION 32

A. TRUE   B. FALSE   C. TRUE   D. FALSE   E. TRUE

QUESTION 33

A. FALSE   B. TRUE   C. TRUE   D. TRUE   E. TRUE

Occlusion of the blood supply to the femoral head can occur in sickle cell disease, caisson disease and Gaucher's disease. Renal transplantation is associated with high steroid intake.

QUESTION 34

A. FALSE   B. TRUE   C. FALSE   D. TRUE   E. TRUE

Ulnar nerve damage results in hypothenar wasting and weakness of thumb adduction. Median nerve damage produces thenar wasting and weakness of thumb abduction and opposition.

QUESTION 35

A. FALSE   B. TRUE   C. TRUE   D. TRUE   E. FALSE

Girls are more commonly affected in the UK. Failure of conservative management or late diagnosis requires surgical management.

QUESTION 36

A. FALSE   B. TRUE   C. FALSE   D. TRUE   E. FALSE

Achalasia is due to impaired peristalsis in the distal oesophagus characterised by the absence of ganglion cells. Carcinoma occurs in 3% of cases. SLE is associated with CREST syndrome, resulting in sclerosis of the oesophagus.

QUESTION 37

A. TRUE   B. FALSE   C. TRUE   D. FALSE   E. TRUE

Portal hypertension may be pre-, intra-, or post- hepatic in aetiology. Collateral circulation develops via oesophago-gastric, ano-rectal and umbilical plexuses. Ascites, hypopoteinaemia and encephalopathy later develop.

QUESTION 38

A. FALSE   B. TRUE   C. FALSE   D. TRUE   E. TRUE

Excessive disease resulting in small bowel resection may give rise to short gut syndrome in adults. The most common cause is Crohn's disease, but any pathology requiring extensive surgery may be responsible.

QUESTION 39

A. FALSE   B. TRUE   C. TRUE   D. FALSE   E. TRUE

Gonococcal strictures are most common at the bulbous urethra. The age of presentation is typically in a younger age group than for prostatic symptoms.

QUESTION 40

A. TRUE   B. FALSE   C. TRUE   D. TRUE   E. FALSE

Also known as a Grawitz tumour and hypernephroma, arises from the renal cortex. It can secrete erythropoetin and other hormones. Spread is primarily blood to the lung and bones, and to local lymph nodes.

QUESTION 41

A. FALSE   B. FALSE   C. TRUE   D. FALSE   E. FALSE

QUESTION 42

A. FALSE   B. TRUE   C. FALSE   D. TRUE   E. FALSE

Medullary carcinoma of the thyroid develops from the parafollicular (C–Cells) which secrete various peptide hormones including calcitonin as well as prostoglandins, 5-HT, ACTH and the tumour marker CEA. Spread is usually via lymphatics and blood to distant sites.

QUESTION 43

A. FALSE   B. FALSE   C. TRUE   D. FALSE   E. TRUE

Carcinoid tumours are derived from the APUD cells (amine precursor uptake decarboxylase) and secrete sertonin (5-hydroxytryptamine) amongst other hormones. The appendix and distal small bowel are the most common sites of origin, but they can occur anywhere along the GI tract and also in the ovaries and bronchi. Five year survival with hepatic metastases is approximately 20%.

QUESTION 44

A. TRUE   B. TRUE   C. TRUE   D. FALSE   E. FALSE

QUESTION 45

A. TRUE B. FALSE C. FALSE D. FALSE E. FALSE

Hormone receptor presence confers a survival advantage. Invasive ductal carcinoma has the worst type prognosis

QUESTION 46

A. FALSE B. TRUE C. FALSE D. FALSE E. TRUE

These lesions resemble sarcoma, and are invasive in 15% of cases. Spread in these situations is via the blood stream to the lung and bones. Local lymph node spread is rare. Treatment is with wide excision or mastectomy.

QUESTION 47

A. FALSE B. TRUE C. TRUE D. FALSE E. TRUE

QUESTION 48

A. FALSE B. TRUE C. TRUE D. FALSE E. TRUE

Babies present with conjugated hyperbilirubinaemia. Type I is limited to the common bile duct. Other GI anomalies include polysplenia and situs inversus

QUESTION 49

A. FALSE B. TRUE C. TRUE D. FALSE E. TRUE

The neural crest cells develop as part of the sympathetic nervous system, and therefore tumours can occur at any point along the extent of the sympathetic chain, and can secrete catecholamines. The tumour can metastasize to bone, liver and skin.

QUESTION 50

A. FALSE B. TRUE C. FALSE D. TRUE E. TRUE